Pocket Handbook
of Esophageal Disorders

Nina Bandyopadhyay · Ronnie Fass
Takahisa Yamasaki · Colin Hemond

Pocket Handbook of Esophageal Disorders

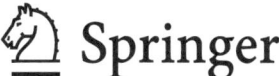

Nina Bandyopadhyay
Digestive Disease Associates Ltd
Wyomissing, PA
USA

Ronnie Fass
The Esophageal and
Swallowing Center, Division
of Gastroenterology
& Hepatology, MetroHealth
Medical Center
Case Western Reserve
University
Cleveland, OH
USA

Takahisa Yamasaki
The Esophageal and
Swallowing Center, Division
of Gastroenterology
& Hepatology, MetroHealth
Medical Center
Case Western Reserve
University
Cleveland, OH
USA

Colin Hemond
The Esophageal and
Swallowing Center, Division
of Gastroenterology
& Hepatology, MetroHealth
Medical Center
Case Western Reserve
University
Cleveland, OH
USA

ISBN 978-3-319-97330-2   ISBN 978-3-319-97331-9   (eBook)
https://doi.org/10.1007/978-3-319-97331-9

Library of Congress Control Number: 2018957087

© Springer Nature Switzerland AG 2019

This work is subject to copyright. All rights are reserved by the Publisher, whether the whole or part of the material is concerned, specifically the rights of translation, reprinting, reuse of illustrations, recitation, broadcasting, reproduction on microfilms or in any other physical way, and transmission or information storage and retrieval, electronic adaptation, computer software, or by similar or dissimilar methodology now known or hereafter developed.

The use of general descriptive names, registered names, trademarks, service marks, etc. in this publication does not imply, even in the absence of a specific statement, that such names are exempt from the relevant protective laws and regulations and therefore free for general use.

The publisher, the authors, and the editors are safe to assume that the advice and information in this book are believed to be true and accurate at the date of publication. Neither the publisher nor the authors or the editors give a warranty, express or implied, with respect to the material contained herein or for any errors or omissions that may have been made. The publisher remains neutral with regard to jurisdictional claims in published maps and institutional affiliations.

This Springer imprint is published by the registered company Springer Nature Switzerland AG
The registered company address is: Gewerbestrasse 11, 6330 Cham, Switzerland

To my wife, Shira, and our children, Ofer, Hagar, and Sharon – for your support and unconditional love all these years.

Ronnie Fass

Preface

This esophageal disorder textbook comes at a time when students, trainees, and busy practicing physicians are interested in an educational resource that is easily accessible, is up to date, and provides state-of-the-art information on the topic but, at the same time, is not too exhaustive and easy to explore. Consequently, Nina, Taka, Colin, and myself have put together a book that is easy to peruse and identify the requested topic, filled with tables, figures, and photos and easy to carry from the office to clinic. The language of the book is easy to understand and the reading relatively fast.

The esophageal disorder field has markedly changed in the last decade, with numerous important developments in the areas of pathophysiology, diagnosis, and management. There was the introduction of new diagnostic techniques in the areas like gastroesophageal reflux disease (GERD), esophageal motor disorders, Barrett's esophagus, eosinophilic esophagitis, and esophageal cancer. There were major developments in the understanding of the pathophysiology of GERD, in particular refractory heartburn, functional esophageal disorders, eosinophilic esophagitis, and esophageal malignancy. In addition, there were many exciting new discoveries in the management of GERD, dysphagia, esophageal motility disorders, eosinophilic esophagitis, and Barrett's esophagus. The introduction of the Rome IV criteria changed the definition of all functional esophageal disorders, which affected the definition of some of the GERD phenotypes. A new functional esophageal disorder, termed "reflux hypersensitivity," was added. One of the areas that have vastly expanded over the last decade was GERD, with the introduction of new diagnostic tools, new medications, several therapeutic endoscopic techniques, and new surgical interventions.

In this book, we cover 15 topics in esophageal disorders, which include esophageal anatomy and physiology, dysphagia, esophageal motility disorders, esophageal manifestations of dermatological conditions, esophageal malignancy, esophageal rings and webs, esophageal diverticula, vascular abnormalities of the esophagus, gastroesophageal reflux disease, functional esophageal disorders, esophageal injury, graft versus host disease, eosinophilic esophagitis, and other esophageal disorders.

As with other books that I was involved with their development, my hope is that this book will be used by students, residents, fellows, other trainees, and physicians from different areas, like primary care, internal medicine, gastroenterology, surgery, and others, for daily clinical purposes related to esophageal disorders and will serve as a first-line educational resource.

Wyomissing, PA, USA	Nina Bandyopadhyay
Cleveland, OH, USA	Ronnie Fass
Cleveland, OH, USA	Takahisa Yamasaki
Cleveland, OH, USA	Colin Hemond

Contents

1. Introduction 1
2. Esophageal Anatomy and Physiology 3
3. Dysphagia 11
4. Esophageal Motility Disorders 17
5. Esophageal Manifestations of Dermatological Conditions 41
6. Esophageal Malignancy 47
7. Rings and Webs 63
8. Esophageal Diverticula 67
9. Vascular Abnormalities of the Esophagus 75
10. Foreign Bodies 77
11. Gastroesophageal Reflux Disease (GERD) 85
12. Functional Esophageal Disorders 123
13. Esophageal Injury 133

14 Graft Versus Host Disease.................... 143

15 Eosinophilic Esophagitis (EoE) 145

16 Other Esophageal Disorders.................... 151

Index 153

Chapter 1
Introduction

The esophagus is a muscular tube connecting the pharynx to the stomach. Although simple in design, the esophagus is a complex organ, the site of a variety of conditions commonly encountered in clinical gastroenterology. Its location and relationships to other aspects of the gastrointestinal tract and thoracic organs make it unique. A complete understanding of this organ is essential for the practicing gastroenterologist.

Chapter 2
Esophageal Anatomy and Physiology

Introduction

Strictly speaking, the esophagus begins with the upper esophageal sphincter (the cricopharyngeus); however, from a functional standpoint, it begins more proximally. The oral cavity and pharynx are critically involved in the process of swallowing. The lips, oral cavity, palate, mandible, and tongue are the components responsible for mastication, bolus formation, and the beginning process of digestion. The food bolus must not only be broken up, but it must also be contained and not allowed to enter the respiratory tract.

Esophageal Anatomy

Strictly speaking, the esophagus begins with the upper esophageal sphincter (the cricopharyngeus); however, from a functional standpoint, it begins more proximally. The oral cavity and pharynx are critically involved in the process of swallowing. The lips, oral cavity, palate, mandible, and tongue are the components responsible for mastication, bolus formation, and the beginning process of digestion. The food bolus must not only be broken up, but it must also be contained and not allowed to enter the respiratory tract.

From the oral cavity, a food bolus enters the oropharynx, which is composed of the base of the tongue anteriorly and the superior, middle, and inferior pharyngeal constrictors posteriorly. At the level of the hypopharynx reside the larynx and the cricopharyngeus. The larynx is suspended in a manner that allows it to be raised and covered by the epiglottis as a bolus of food is traversing the pharynx. The movement is essential to the act of swallowing and protecting of the airway.

The cricopharyngeus is a skeletal muscle sphincter, which separates the pharynx from the tubular esophagus. This sphincter is radially asymmetrical, exerting maximal force in the anterior-posterior axis. It is innervated by the pharyngeal branch of the vagus nerve. The tubular esophagus begins after the cricopharyngeus and consists of a muscular tube averaging 20–22 cm in length (range 17–30 cm). The esophagus is composed of skeletal muscle proximally and smooth muscle

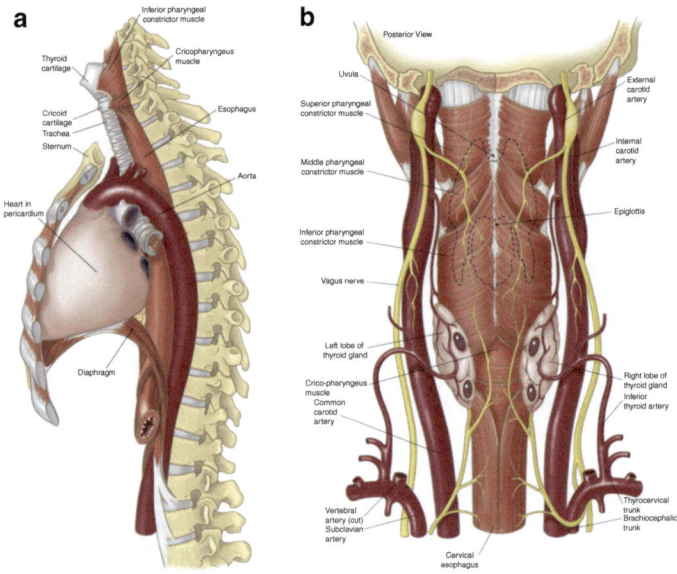

FIGURE 2.1 Esophageal anatomy. (**a**) The esophagus descends anteriorly to the vertebral column through the middle mediastinum and traverses the diaphragmatic hiatus into the abdomen at the level of the tenth thoracic vertebral body. (**b**) Posterior view of the pharynx and cervical esophagus. (With permission from Oezcelik and DeMeester [1])

distally (see Fig. 2.1) [1]. Autopsy studies suggest that the proximal 5% of the tubular esophagus are skeletal muscle, the middle 35–40% are mixed, and the distal 50–60% are smooth muscle. The muscular layers of the esophagus are arranged in circular and longitudinal bundles. The esophagus has no serosal layer. Situated between the muscular layers is the myenteric plexus. The submucosal or Meissner's plexus is found between the circular layer and the muscularis mucosae (see Fig. 2.2) [2]. The ganglia of the myenteric plexus are more prominent in the smooth muscle areas of the tubular esophagus and are thought to integrate messages from the vagus to the muscles of the esophagus.

At the junction of the esophagus and stomach is the lower esophageal sphincter (LES). Historically, the LES was considered as a physiological sphincter without a clear anatomic structure. Current data suggests that the LES is principally composed of circular muscle of the distal 2–3 cm of the esophagus and the oblique muscle fibers running from the lesser curvature to the greater curvature, the gastric sling

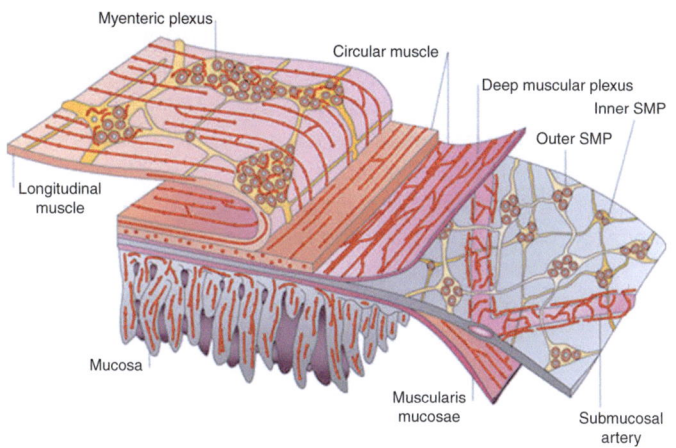

FIGURE 2.2 The enteric nervous system of the esophagus. The esophagus has two main ganglionated plexuses: the myenteric plexus, located between the muscular layers, and the submucosal plexus which is found between the circular layer and the muscularis mucosae. *SMP* submucosal plexus. (With permission from Furness [2])

fibers. The right crus of the diaphragm support the LES in its function as a barrier by physically encircling it and providing mechanical support, particularly during physical exertion.

Physiology of Swallowing

The process of swallowing is complex and requires fine coordination involving multiple muscle groups. The progress begins with the heavily innervated tongue and pharynx. The trigeminal, facial and glossopharyngeal, vagus and hypoglossal nerves innervate the pharyngeal muscles. Vagal neurons controlling the pharynx and skeletal muscle of the esophagus originate from the nucleus ambiguous. Although the smooth muscle portions of the tubular esophagus are innervated by the vagus nerve – and it's the vagus nerve that controls peristalsis under physiological conditions – peristalsis in this portion of the esophagus will continue, even if the vagal innervation is removed. The neural plexuses of the smooth muscle esophagus control its activity via excitation of the circular and longitudinal muscle bundles by muscarinic receptors or inhibition of the circular muscle layer by noradrenergic, noncholinergic neurotransmitters, nitric oxide (NO), and vasoactive intestinal polypeptide (VIP). Swallowing begins when the food bolus propels into the pharynx from the mouth. In rapid sequence and with precise coordination, the larynx is elevated, and the epiglottis seals the airway. The upper esophageal sphincter relaxes, and the bolus moves into the tubular esophagus. Peristaltic pressures are generated ranging from 40 to 180 mmHg. The measured pressures tend to be lower in the more proximal portions of the esophagus and higher in the distal smooth muscle portion of the esophagus. Pressures will vary not only by location but also by consistency (i.e., solid or highly viscous boluses require greater pressure), volume, and temperature of the bolus itself. Movement through the tubular esophagus is controlled by the vagus nerve, concomitantly with the initiation of a swallow. The LES relaxes to gastric baseline immediately with swallowing initiation. As bolus moves distally, the LES remains relaxed (deglutitive inhibition). Once the bolus enters into the stomach, the LES returns to its state of tonic contraction preventing movement of gastric content back into the esophagus.

The LES is a 2–3 cm segment of the tonically contracted smooth muscle at the esophagogastric junction. It is believed that the tonic contraction of this portion of the esophagus is a function of the muscle itself and not dependent on the neural innervation. Stimulation of the inhibitory fibers results in LES relaxation. The resting tone of the LES is typically between 10 and 45 mmHg and is affected by a wide array of events, foods, drugs, and hormones. LES relaxation occurs not only in response to swallowing but also in response to esophageal distension and fundic distension by balloon or meal and may even occur without prior primary or secondary peristalsis. LES relaxation without prior peristaltic wave is referred to as a transient lower esophageal sphincter relaxation (TLESR) and is considered a normal part of esophageal function. It is a vagally mediated reflex triggered by fundic distension and the mechanism responsive for belching. TLESRs play an integral role in almost all gastroesophageal reflux episodes in healthy subjects and most (55–80%) reflux episodes in patients with GERD. Factors affecting the rate of TLESRs include pharyngeal stimulation and cholecystokinin. In addition, sleep, anesthesia, and supine position mediate inhibition of TLESRs. Substances shown to inhibit TLESR events include cholecystokinin A (CCKA) antagonists, anticholinergic agents (e.g., atropine), nitric oxide synthase inhibitors, morphine, and gamma-aminobutyric acid B (GABA-B) agonists (e.g., baclofen).

Esophageal Sensory Innervation

The esophagus, like the rest of the visceral organs, receives dual sensory innervation, traditionally referred to as a parasympathetic and sympathetic but properly based on actual nerves, vagal and spinal. The vagal afferent neurons compose

80% of the vagal trunk and have cell bodies in the nodose ganglia. Vagal afferents, whose receptive fields are located in the esophageal smooth muscle layer, are sensitive to mechanical distension, while polymodal (responding to multiple modalities of stimuli) vagal afferents with receptive fields between the muscularis mucosae and propria are sensitive to a variety of chemical or mechanical intraluminal stimuli which, under normal circumstances, are not associated with conscious perception. Recent data indicate that vagal afferents do respond to nociceptive stimuli, which include alpha, beta-methylene ATP, 5-hydroxytryptamine (serotonin), and capsaicin or bile topically applied to the esophageal mucosa. In contrast, spinal afferents, which have their cell bodies in the dorsal root ganglion, are primary acting as nociceptors and are central to the perception of discomfort and pain. Spinal afferents with receptive fields in the muscle layer are primarily mechanosensitive. The intraepithelial nerve endings of the spinal afferents are likely to be involved in mediating acid-induced pain during topical exposure to intraluminal acid. Many of the afferents contain calcitonin gene-related peptide and substance P, neurotransmitters that are important in mediating visceral nociception.

Data regarding cortical loci involved in the process of esophageal sensation in humans are relatively scarce. Non-painful esophageal balloon distensions elicit bilateral activation along the central sulcus, insular cortex, and the frontal and parietal operculum. In contrast, painful esophageal balloon distension results in intense activation of the same areas and additional activation of the right anterior cingulate cortex (important in affective processing) and anterior cingulate gyrus (important in pain processing and generating an affective and cognitive response to pain). Non-painful infusion of 0.1 N hydrochloric acid results in cerebral cortical activity that was concentrated in the posterior cingulate, the parietal and anteromesial frontal lobes. The superior frontal lobe regions activated corresponded to Brodmann's area 32, the insula, the operculum, and anterior cingulate.

References

1. Oezcelik A, DeMeester SR. General anatomy of the esophagus. Thorac Surg Clin. 2011;21:289–97.
2. Furness JB. The enteric nervous system and neurogastroenterology. Nat Rev Gastroenterol Hepatol. 2012;9:286–94.

Chapter 3
Dysphagia

Introduction

Dysphagia means difficulty in swallowing. Dysphagia may result from any alteration of the swallowing process from food introduction into the mouth and bolus entry into the stomach. Given the complexity of this process, it is clear that a wide array of mechanical and functional abnormalities may result in dysphagia. Despite the large number of possible etiologies, dysphagia may be divided into abnormalities related to the movement of a food bolus from the mouth and into the esophagus (transfer or oropharyngeal dysphagia) or alterations in the movement of food bolus through the esophagus and entry into the stomach (transport or esophageal dysphagia).

Oropharyngeal Dysphagia

The process of moving a food bolus, in particular liquids, from the mouth to the esophagus, while coming in close proximity to the airway, requires a fine coordination of events happening at a very rapid rate. Patients describe having difficulty in initiating a swallow and usually identify the cervical area as the location of the problem. Other symptoms attributed to oropharyngeal dysphagia include the sensation of food sticking immediately upon swallowing, often with choking, coughing, or nasal regurgitation. Disruption of this phase of swallowing may be commonly caused by neuromuscular dysfunction and structural defects as well as other causes. See Table 3.1 for comprehensive review of etiologies for oropharyngeal dysphagia [1]. Structural abnormalities that may be encountered in the hypopharynx include cervical osteophytes, hypopharyngeal diverticulum (Zenker's diverticulum), head and neck tumors, radiation-induced changes, or post-cricoid webs. In these settings, patients may also note difficulties in moving a solid food bolus from the mouth and into the tubular esophagus.

Much more commonly, symptoms of transfer dysphagia are the result of neuromuscular injury resulting in the disruption of the finely coordinated act of swallowing. In these situations, problems are much more commonly associated with attempts to swallow liquids. Both sensory and motor injuries may result in an inability to accomplish the transfer of a bolus from the mouth to the esophagus. Young patients with oropharyngeal dysphagia more often have etiologies related to muscle disease, webs, or rings, while older patients more commonly have stroke, dementia, and Parkinson's disease. Stroke is one of the most common causes of oropharyngeal dysphagia and commonly is seen with both brain stem and cortical types of strokes. The presence of dysphagia in the setting of a stroke is associated with a high patient mortality related to a higher risk of aspiration pneumonia and dehydration.

Essentially, any disease process that affects the brain can result in dysphagia. The more common associations are amyotrophic lateral sclerosis, Parkinson's disease, and brain tumors. Primary muscular disease may also result in oropharyngeal dysphagia. These include oculopharyngeal muscular dystrophy, myotonic dystrophy, myasthenia gravis, and tardive dyskinesia. Swallowing impairment often leads to decreased oral intake and ultimately malnutrition, depression, and isolation.

Table 3.1 Etiologies for oropharyngeal dysphagia

Neurologic diseases	Metabolic diseases	Structural diseases
Cerebrovascular accident	Hyperthyroidism	Inflammatory (pharyngitis, abscess, tuberculosis)
Parkinson disease		Congenital webs
Multiple sclerosis	*Inflammatory/autoimmune diseases*	Plummer-Vinson syndrome
Brain neoplasm	Amyloidosis	Neoplasm
Polio and post–polio syndrome	Sarcoidosis	Cricopharyngeal bar
Alzheimer disease	Systemic lupus erythematosus	Zenker diverticulum
Huntington disease		Extrinsic compression (osteophytes, goiter, lymphadenopathy)
	Infectious diseases	Bullous skin diseases
Myopathic diseases	Meningitis	Poor dentition
Myositis	Diphtheria	
Dermatomyositis	Botulism	*Iatrogenic diseases*
Myasthenia gravis	Lyme disease	Medication side effects (neuroleptics)
Muscular dystrophies	Syphilis	Surgical resection
	Viral (coxsackie, herpes, cytomegalovirus)	Radiation-induced
		Corrosive (pill-injury, intentional)

With permission from Gasiorowska and Fass [1]

Major diagnostic tests for oropharyngeal dysphagia include modified barium swallow, nasoendoscopy, fiberoptic endoscopic evaluation of swallow (FEES), and pharyngeal high-resolution manometry. In addition, patients should undergo a full evaluation by speech pathology and ENT physician.

Esophageal Dysphagia

Once the food bolus enters the esophagus, structural abnormalities or alterations in esophageal motility may cause resistance to the smooth passage of food through the esophagus and into the stomach. Patients with esophageal dysphagia usually report onset of symptoms several seconds after initiating a swallow and can localize symptoms anywhere along the esophagus. Solid food dysphagia alone is commonly associated with mechanical obstruction, whereas solid and liquid dysphagia are seen in patients with esophageal motility disorders, such as achalasia.

Etiologies for esophageal dysphagia range from congenital abnormalities to acquired conditions, constituting a rather large differential diagnosis (see Table 3.2) [1]. Diagnostic testing to evaluate for esophageal dysphagia includes upper endoscopy, high-resolution esophageal manometry, chest CT, and barium swallow or esophagram.

Table 3.11 Differential diagnoses for esophageal dysphagia

Neuromuscular disorders
Achalasia (all types)
Distal esophageal spasm
Scleroderma
Gastroesophageal reflux disease
Esophagogastric junction outflow obstruction
Ineffective esophageal motility
Absent contractility
Structural lesions (intrinsic)
Benign peptic stricture
Esophageal rings and webs
Esophageal diverticula
Foreign bodies
Esophageal carcinoma
Medication-induced inflammation or strictures
Eosinophilic esophagitis
Structural lesions (extrinsic)
Vascular compression
Mediastinal lesions
Cervical osteoarthritis

With permission from Gasiorowska and Fass [1]

Reference

1. Gasiorowska A, Fass R. Current approach to dysphagia. Gastroenterol Hepatol. 2009;5:269–79.

Chapter 4
Esophageal Motility Disorders

Introduction

The newest iteration of the Chicago Classification, v3.0, was introduced in 2014 and defines esophageal motility disorders as the following: (1) achalasia types I–III; (2) esophagogastric junction outflow obstruction (EGJOO); (3) major disorders of peristalsis, absent contractility, distal esophageal spasm, and hypercontractile esophagus (jackhammer esophagus); and (4) minor disorders of peristalsis, ineffective esophageal motility (IEM) and fragmented peristalsis. See Table 4.1 and Fig. 4.1 for full characterization based on high-resolution esophageal manometry parameters [1].

High-Resolution Esophageal Manometry

High-resolution esophageal manometry (HREM) has replaced conventional esophageal manometry in defining esophageal motility. HREM is composed of a catheter with several closely spaced sensors that measure esophageal pressures. The data can be translated into pressure topography plots (Clouse plots) of spatiotemporal pressure points along the esophagus. The integrated relaxation pressure (IRP) is the lowest mean esophagogastric junction pressure for 4 s during swallowing (normal median IRP <15 mmHg).

TABLE 4.1 The Chicago Classification of esophageal motility v3.0. Definitions of esophageal motility disorders as per Chicago Classification v3.0 were divided into types of achalasia and EGJ outflow obstruction, major and minor disorders of peristalsis

Esophageal Motor disorder	Criteria
Achalasia and EGJ Outflow Obstruction	Elevated median IRP (>15 mmHg[a]), 100% failed peristalsis
Type I achalasia (classic achalasia)	(DCI <100 mmHg)
	Premature contractions with DCI values less than 450 mmHg·s·cm satisfy criteria for failed peristalsis
Type II achalasia (with esophageal compression)	Elevated median IRP (>15 mmHg[a]), 100% failed peristalsis, panesophageal pressurization with ≥20% of swallows
	Contractions may be masked by esophageal pressurization and DCI should not be calculated
Type III achalasia (spastic achalasia)	Elevated median IRP (>15 mmHg[a]), no normal peristalsis, premature (spastic) contractions with DCI >450 mmHg·s·cm with ≥20% of swallows
	May be mixed with panesophageal pressurization
EGJ outflow obstruction	Elevated median IRP (>15 mmHg[a]), sufficient evidence of peristalsis such that criteria for types I-III achalasia are not met[b]
Major disorders of peristalsis	*(Not encountered in normal subjects)*
Absent contractility	Normal median IRP, 100% failed peristalsis
	Achalasia should be considered when IRP values are borderline and when there is evidence of esophageal pressurization

TABLE 4.1 (continued)

Esophageal Motor disorder	Criteria
	Premature contractions with DCI values less than 450 mmHg·s·cm *meet criteria for failed peristalsis*
Distal esophageal spasm	Normal median IRP, ≥20% premature contractions with DCI >450 mmHg·s·cm[a]. Some normal peristalsis may be present
Hypercontractile esophagus (jackhammer)	At least two swallows with DCI >8000 mmHg·s·cm[a],[c]
	Hypercontractility may involve, or even be localized to, the LES
Minor disorders of peristalsis	*(Characterized by contractile vigor and contraction pattern)*
Ineffective esophageal motility (IEM)	≥50% ineffective swallows
	Ineffective swallows can be failed or weak (DCI <450 mmHg·s·cm)
	Multiple repetitive swallow assessment may be helpful in determining peristaltic reserve
Fragmented peristalsis	≥50% fragmented contractions with DCI >450 mmHg·s·cm
Normal esophageal motility	Not fulfilling any of the above classifications

With permission from Kahrilas et al. [1]
[a]Cutoff value dependent on the manometric hardware; this is the cutoff for the Sierra device
[b]Potential etiologies: early achalasia, mechanical obstruction, esophageal wall stiffness, or manifestation of hiatal hernia
[c]Hypercontractile esophagus can be a manifestation of outflow obstruction as evident by instances in which it occurs in association with an IRP greater than the upper limit of normal

Chapter 4. Esophageal Motility Disorders

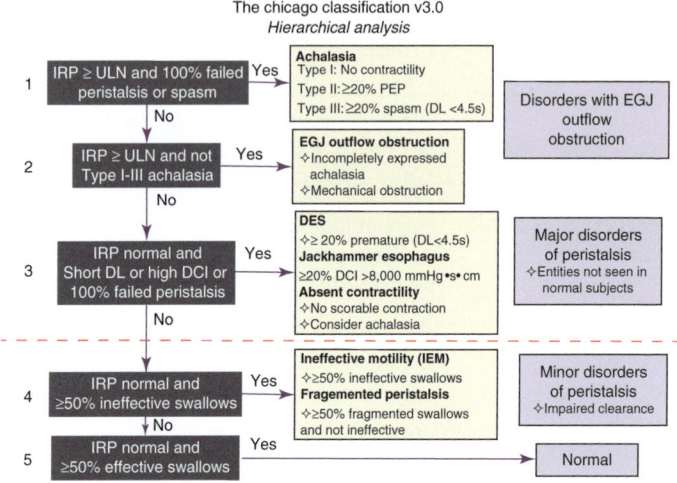

FIGURE 4.1 Hierarchical algorithm for the interpretation of esophageal HRM studies with Chicago Classification v3.0. Diagnostic algorithm to aid in the diagnosis of esophageal motility disorders according to the Chicago Classification v3.0. (With permission from Kahrilas et al. [1])

The IRP has replaced the LES relaxation residual pressure obtained previously on conventional manometry. The contractile deceleration point (CDP) is defined as the point at which peristalsis stops and the esophagus begins to empty. The distal latency (DL) measures the time from the start of the swallow to the CDP (normal DL >4.5 s). The distal contractile integral (DCI) measures the vigor of the smooth muscle peristaltic contraction.

When evaluating patterns of esophageal contractility using high-resolution manometry topographic information, three parameters are evaluated: contraction vigor, contraction pattern, and intrabolus pressure pattern. The vigor of contractions is characterized as normal (DCI >450 mmHg·s·cm), failed (DCI <100 mmHg·s·cm), weak (<450 mmHg·s·cm), and hypercontractile (DCI ≥8000 mmHg·s·cm). Contraction patterns are described as premature if DL is <4.5 s or fragmented if breaks in esophageal peristalsis are >5 cm in length within the 20 mmHg isobaric contour with DCI >450 mmHg. Intrabolus pressure patterns describe pan esophageal pressurization (pressurization >30 mmHg extending uniformly between the UES and LES), compartmentalized esophageal pressure of >30 mmHg extending from contractile front to EGJ and EGJ pressurization, which is seen only between the LES and crural diaphragm along with separate pressure patterns for the LES and crural diaphragm.

Primary Esophageal Motility Disorders

This term refers to a number of conditions in which there is a disruption in the neuromuscular control of esophageal peristalsis that is not driven by a systemic disorder.

Achalasia

The phenotype of esophageal dysmotility is achalasia and is considered one of the most widely recognized primary esophageal motility disorder. This condition, characterized by loss of esophageal peristalsis and failure of LES relaxation, is thought to be related to loss or decreased number of myenteric neurons in the esophagus. Accumulating data point to viral infection, in genetically susceptible individuals, to cause an aberrant immune response leading to ganglionitis and subsequent esophageal neuron loss. Additional changes have been described in patients with this condition: (1) loss of ganglion cells from the myenteric plexus; (2) degenerative changes in the vagus nerve; (3) degenerative changes in the dorsal motor nucleus of the vagus, including occasional evidence of intracytoplasmic inclusions (Lewy small nerve fiber bodies); (4) loss of small intramuscular nerve fibers; (5) reduction in vesicles; and (6) HLA DQA1 *0103 allele and HLA DQB1*0603 allele associated with antibodies against myenteric neurons in patients with achalasia.

Achalasia may occur at any age from childhood to late adulthood. The peak occurrence is between the ages 30 and 60 years, with increased incidence with older age. The mean incidence is 0.3–1.63 per 100,000 with a mean prevalence of 8.7–10.7 per 100,000. Familial clusters among siblings have been described. Men and women have equal incidence, with no racial preference. Achalasia may also be seen as a complication of Chagas disease – a parasitic infection with protozoa *Trypanosoma cruzi* – as well as malignant lesions (pseudoachalasia), the latter of which has been associated with adenocarcinoma of the cardia and paraneoplastic small-cell lung cancer (positive anti-Hu antibody). Additionally, achalasia can be seen in association with autoimmune conditions such as type I diabetes mellitus, hypothyroidism, Sjogren's disease and uveitis, Allgrove syndrome (e.g., triple-A syndrome), Down syndrome, familial visceral neuropathy, as well as degenerative neurological conditions such as Parkinson's disease, neurofibromatosis, and hereditary cerebellar ataxia. Recently, achalasia types 2 and 3 have been shown to be a complication of opiates consumption.

Patients experience symptoms which are related to impaired transit of food and secretions into the stomach resulting in stasis in the esophagus and possibly increasing the risk by this way for esophageal adenocarcinoma. The hallmark symptom of achalasia is dysphagia, typically for both solids and liquids. Other commonly noted symptoms include regurgitation of undigested food, respiratory symptoms (nocturnal cough, aspiration, recurrent pneumonia), and weight loss. Symptoms are typically present for years prior to diagnosis, especially if the patients are carefully interviewed. Weight loss may be encountered as well. See Fig. 4.2 for the endoscopic appearance of a patient with achalasia.

Neuronal denervation is the underlying mechanism of achalasia. This results in failure of esophageal body peristalsis and failure of the LES to relax in response to swallowing. In achalasia, the esophagus empties by hydrostatic pressure. Specifically, the height of the column of food/fluid forces opens the tonically closed LES. These features result in gradual dilation of the esophagus, with the development of

Primary Esophageal Motility Disorders 23

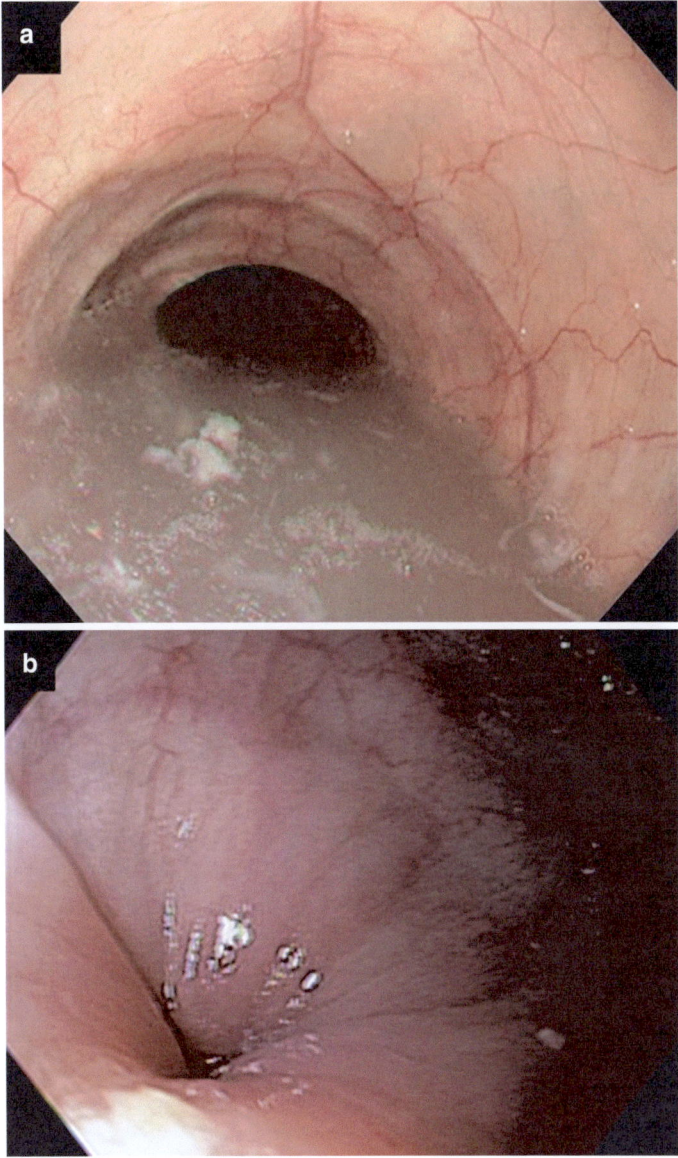

FIGURE 4.2 The endoscopic appearance of patient with achalasia. (**a**) Food residual in the esophagus. (**b**) Stenosis of esophagogastric junction

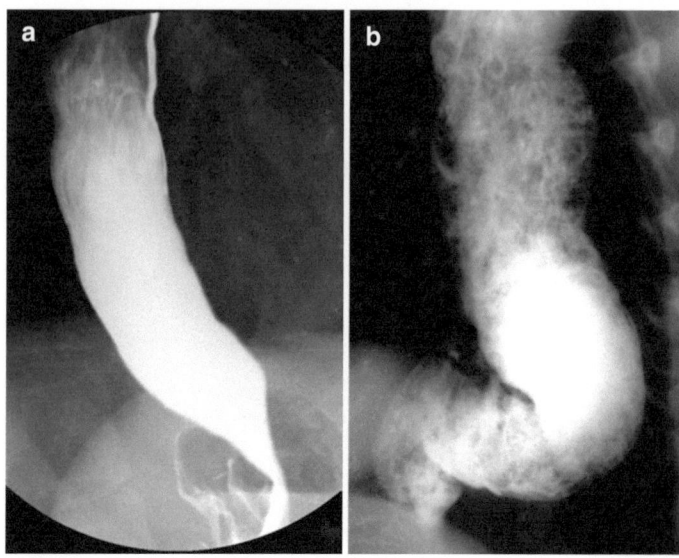

Figure 4.3 Radiographic findings of achalasia. (**a**) Typical bird's beak appearance in early achalasia. (**b**) Sigmoid-like appearance of decompensated esophagus. (With permission from Boeckxstaens et al. [2])

the so-called bird's beak deformity at the LES (diagnosed radiographically) (Fig. 4.3a) [2]. Early cases of achalasia may not exhibit these features. Radiographically, the esophagus will reflect the chronicity of the disease. In early achalasia, the esophagus may appear normal or have a few tertiary contractions. As the disease progresses, the esophagus becomes dilated, and in cases of late diagnosis, the esophagus is so markedly dilated that it assumes a sigmoid configuration (Fig. 4.3b) [2]. In the latter situation, the esophagus rotates to the right, and a right angle is formed between the distal esophagus and the LES. This makes a blind passage of a manometry catheter or balloon dilator difficult and sometimes risky.

Esophageal manometry is often used to confirm the diagnosis of achalasia. The hallmark features are (1) aperistalsis,

(2) hypertensive LES (variably seen), (3) lack or incomplete LES relaxation (variably seen), and (4) reversal of the normal gradient across the LES (normally esophageal baseline pressure is lower than intragastric pressure). The first criterion is necessary for the diagnosis of achalasia, while the other criteria are supportive.

High-resolution esophageal manometry identified three subtypes of achalasia, all of which are associated with incomplete LES relaxation as measured by an elevated integrated relaxation pressure (IRP) of >15 mmHg, while the other criteria used to describe the subtype of achalasia. As per the latest Chicago Classification of esophageal motility disorders, the achalasia subtypes are defined as the following: type I (classic achalasia) is characterized by 100% failed peristalsis, type II (with pan pressurization) is associated with 100% failed peristalsis with simultaneous pressurization throughout the esophagus in ≥20% of swallows, and type III (spastic achalasia) is noted to have no normal peristalsis and premature (spastic) contractions, with DCI values >450 mmHg·s·cm of ≥20% of the swallows. See Fig. 4.4 for high-resolution esophageal manometries of achalasia types I, II, and III.

When achalasia is suspected, a barium swallow should be considered. Early in the disease, the esophagus is normal in diameter. As the disease progresses, the esophagus becomes more dilated and tortuous and does not empty, and the retained food and saliva produce an air-fluid level at the top of the barium column. The distal esophagus is characterized by a smooth tapering leading to the closed lower esophageal sphincter, resembling the "bird's beak" appearance. In half of the patients, the gastric bubble under the diaphragm cannot be seen on chest X-ray. All patients with suspected achalasia should have an upper endoscopy to exclude the presence of gastroesophageal junction malignancy. This is of particular importance in elderly patients with history of rapid onset of dysphagia and profound weight loss.

Treatment of achalasia includes (1) medical therapy with nitrates or calcium channel blockers; (2) botulinum toxin injection; (3) pneumatic dilation; (4) myotomy, performed

Chapter 4. Esophageal Motility Disorders

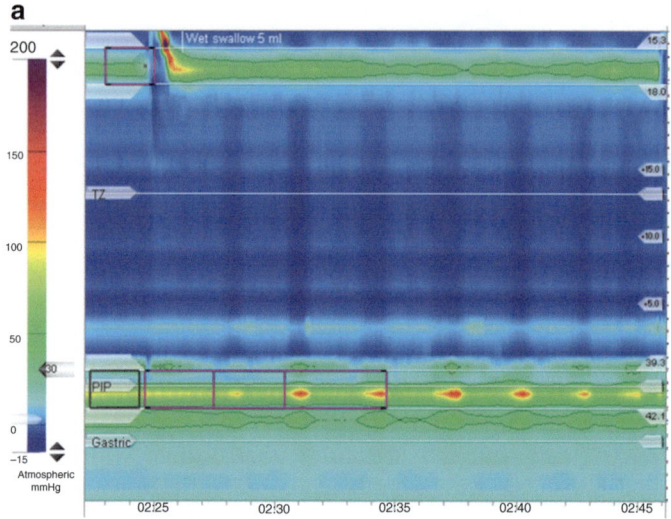

FIGURE 4.4 High-resolution esophageal manometry of patients with achalasia types I, II, and III. These are representative swallows from high-resolution esophageal manometries of three patients with three different patterns of achalasia. All three patients were symptomatic with dysphagia at the time of esophageal manometry. (**a**) Achalasia type I. There is an elevated IRP with no peristalsis noted in the esophagus. IRP = 38, mean resting LES pressure = 77. (**b**) Achalasia type II. This swallow shows the distinctive pattern of pan pressurization, typical of achalasia type II. IRP = 16, mean resting LES pressure = 35. (**c**) Achalasia type III. 20% of swallows in this manometry were noted to have premature contractions. IRP = 26, resting LES pressure 62. *IRP* integrated residual pressure, *LES* lower esophageal sphincter

Primary Esophageal Motility Disorders

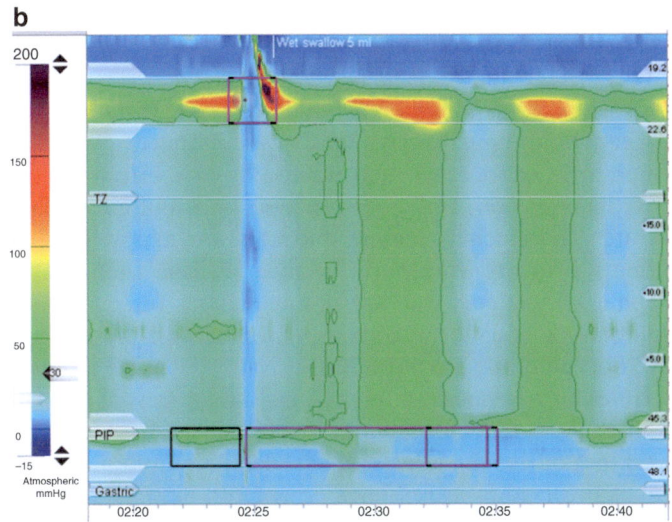

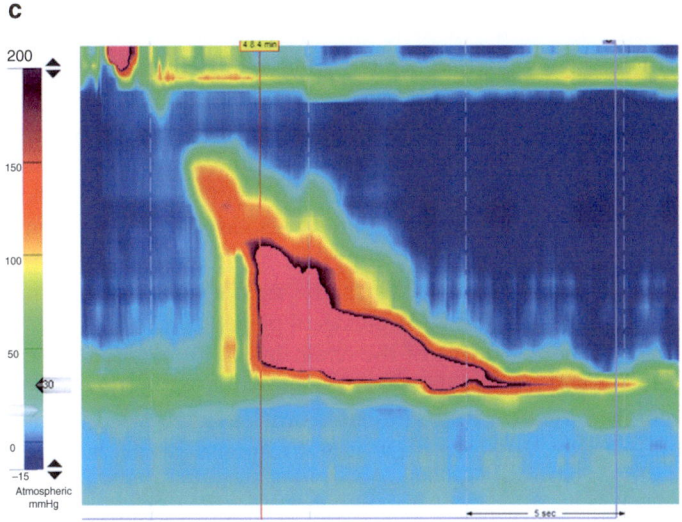

FIGURE 4.4 (continued)

either laparoscopically or in the traditional transthoracic approach (Heller myotomy); (5) peroral endoscopic myotomy (POEM); and (6) esophagectomy.

Pharmacologic treatment with nitrates or calcium channel blockers before meals may improve symptoms of dysphagia temporarily, but treatment is limited by side effects (headache, hypotension, and pedal edema) and limited efficacy. Nitrates and calcium channel blockers are mainly used in patients who are very early in their disease (non-dilated esophagus), patients who are not candidates for pneumatic dilation or surgery, or those who refuse invasive therapy and failed botulinum toxin injections.

Botulinum toxin injection appears to work best in patients older than 50 years. Botulinum toxin A injection is a neurotoxin that blocks the release of acetylcholine from nerve terminals involved in increasing LES smooth muscle tone. The effect of the drug is limited to a period of 6–24 months, at which time retreatment is required (4 quadrant injections just above the esophagogastric junction, totaling 80–100 units).

Pneumatic dilation with a rigid balloon of 30, 35, and 40 mm has been frequently used by gastroenterologists. Results vary, with 50–85% of patients reporting a good to excellent outcome after one dilation. Approximately one third of the patients will relapse after 4–6 years and require additional dilation. Patients with type II achalasia have been found to have the best outcome after pneumatic dilation compared to the other achalasia subtypes. The most serious complication of pneumatic dilation is esophageal perforation, which occurs in 2% (range 0–16%) of the cases. In addition, 15–35% post dilation will report GERD, which improves with proton pump inhibitor therapy. Repeat dilations with a larger sized balloon are usually attempted if the initial response is unsatisfactory. Failure to respond to at least two well-placed balloon dilations is considered by many as a reason for referral to surgery.

The introduction of minimally invasive surgical techniques, either transthoracic or transabdominal, has led some to proceed directly to surgical intervention: longitudinal dissection of muscle fibers of the LES. In a recent meta-analysis of 201 patients, the authors compared the clinical outcomes post pneumatic dilation and Heller myotomy. The results indicated comparable clinical outcomes with both modalities at 43-month follow-up. However, two recent meta-analyses from 2013 indicated superior outcomes with Heller myotomy compared to pneumatic dilation in patients with achalasia.

Complications such as GERD commonly occur after myotomy, and in anticipation of this outcome, myotomy is often done with partial fundoplication (Dor procedure). Esophageal stricture may also occur after myotomy, and incomplete myotomy may lead to recurrent dysphagia. The traditional Heller myotomy has favorable long-term results in 65–85% treated achalasia patients; however, prior therapy with botulinum toxin causes local inflammatory changes which may interfere with surgical intervention.

Peroral endoscopic myotomy (POEM) is a newer endoscopic technique in which a submucosal tunnel is created in the esophageal mucosa below the LES. Subsequently, circular muscle is dissected along 7 cm of the esophagus and 2 cm of the gastric cardia, thereby causing LES disruption. The reported success rates, mostly from small case series, indicate 89–100% improvement of symptoms, even in patients with prior pneumatic dilation. The major side effect of this technique is GERD, because an anti-reflux procedure is not done routinely post POEM. Most patients are placed on anti-reflux medication post POEM.

Approximately 2–5% of the patients develop end-stage achalasia with massive dilation of the esophagus and food retention. These patients are at increased risk of squamous cell carcinoma of the esophagus. Esophagectomy is offered to these patients to improve quality of life and to eliminate the risk of esophageal cancer.

Secondary Achalasia

A variety of conditions may result in a syndrome resembling achalasia. The most common is malignancy, often at the gastroesophageal junction (adenocarcinoma of the cardia, gastric lymphoma, etc.) but, in some cases, distant from this area (small-cell lung cancer, Hodgkin's lymphoma, hepatocellular carcinoma, etc.). Secondary achalasia produces a syndrome that radiographically and manometrically is indistinguishable from primary achalasia. In addition, it is typically seen in older patients in whom the development of dysphagia is rapid. Most cases will be identified by performing endoscopic examination. Other disorders, which may present with an achalasia-like pattern, include Chagas disease (South American trypanosomiasis), intestinal pseudo-obstruction, tight surgical fundoplication, etc.

Absent Contractility

Absent contractility is defined by the presence of 100% failed peristalsis (DCI <100 mmHg·s·cm) in patients with normal IRP. Premature contractions with DCI values that are <450 mmHg·s·cm are considered to meet the criteria for failed peristalsis. See Fig. 4.5a for high-resolution esophageal manometry of absent contractility. The pathogenesis is not well understood, but it has been associated with systemic disorders such as scleroderma, mixed connective tissue disorder, and amyloidosis. In patients with absent contractility, but with borderline IRP values, achalasia type I should be excluded. Absent contractility has been seen in patients with severe GERD, although direction of causality is unclear. Patients with absent contractility are more prone to develop GERD-related complications, such as advance grading of erosive esophagitis, peptic stricture, and Barrett's esophagus. There are no pharmacological modalities that have been proven to restore esophageal peristalsis. Patients are often advised of lifestyle and dietary modifications in order to decrease the risk of bolus retention. These include food lubrication with gravy, dressing, or sauce, sitting upright while eating a meal at least 3–4 h before lying down, drinking warm fluid with food, and drinking room temperature carbonated

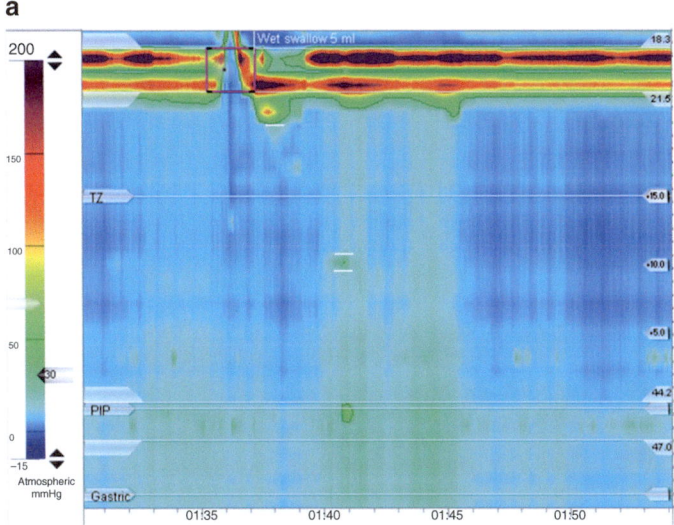

FIGURE 4.5 Examples of high-resolution esophageal manometries of patients with esophageal motor disorders, as per Chicago Classification version 3.0. These are patients diagnosed with (**a**) absent contractility. There is 100% failed esophageal peristalsis noted on this swallow with a normal IRP. IRP = 2, DCI = 0. (**b**) Distal esophageal spasm. The peristaltic wave is noted to have DCI of 1708, normal IRP of 12, with premature contraction (DL = 3.6). (**c**) Jackhammer esophagus. DCI = 14,920, IRP = 15. (**d**) EGJ outflow obstruction. Patient with IRP of 35, with normal peristaltic wave. DCI = 1600. DL = 6.4. (**e**) Ineffective esophageal motility. Low amplitude peristaltic wave noted in the esophagus with normal IRP, DCI of 121, DL = 6.4. *IRP* integrated residual pressure, *DCI* distal contractile integral, *DL* distal latency

32 Chapter 4. Esophageal Motility Disorders

b

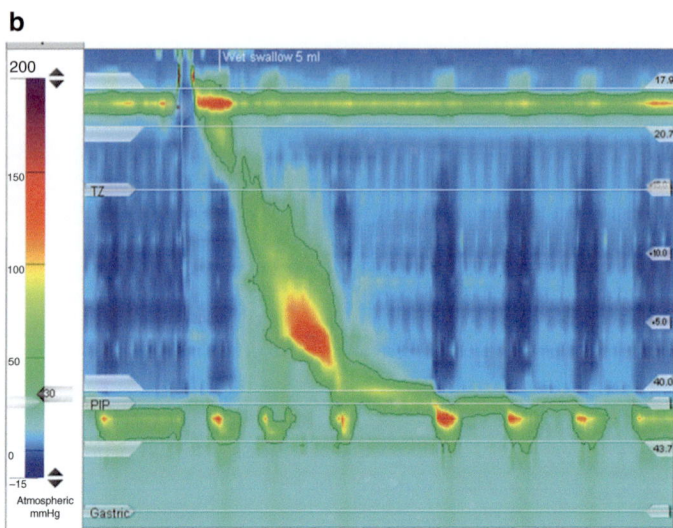

c

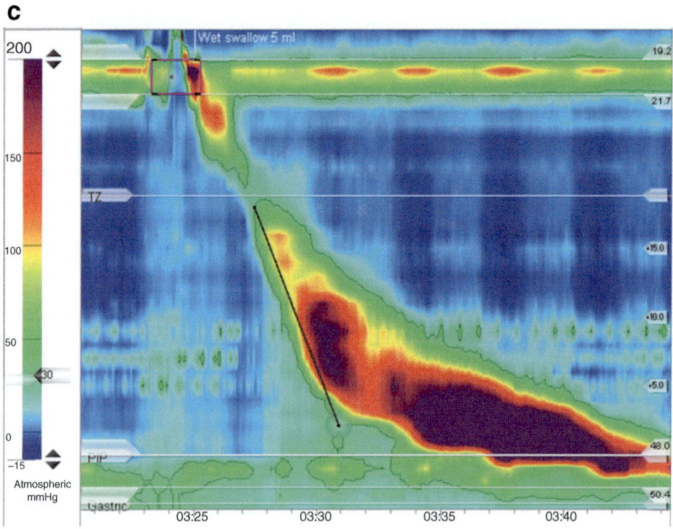

FIGURE 4.5 (continued)

Primary Esophageal Motility Disorders 33

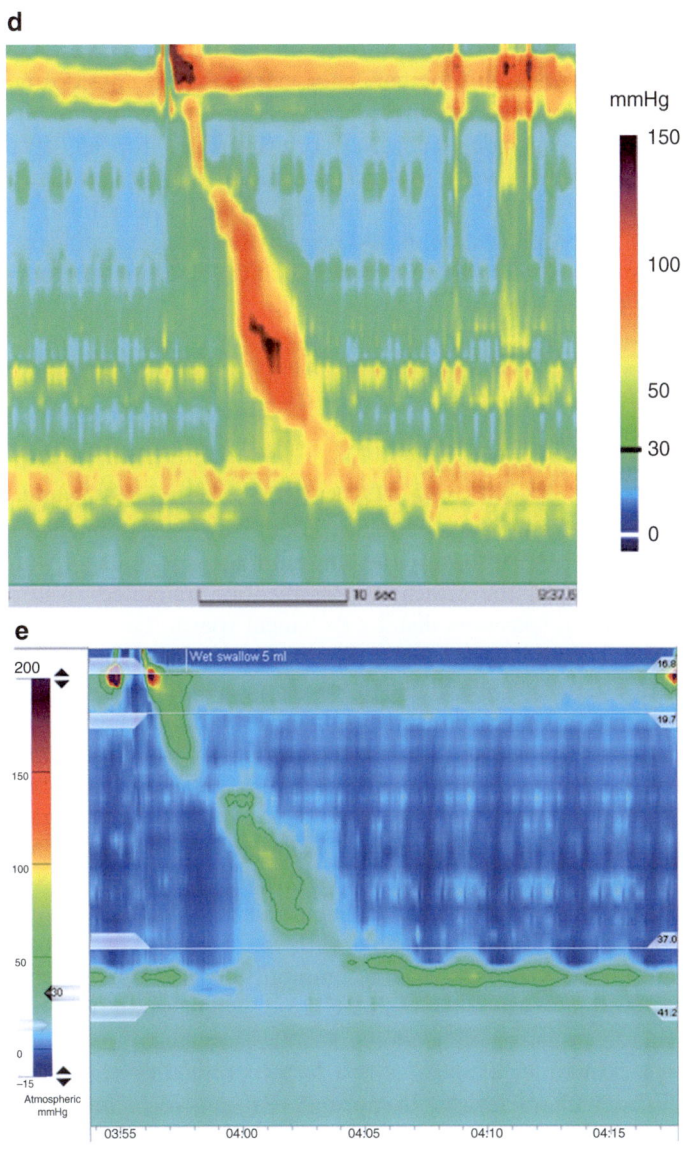

FIGURE 4.5 (continued)

beverages. In addition, aggressive treatment of GERD is highly recommended. A variety of medications have been proposed, including bethanechol, edrophonium, pyridostigmine, domperidone, metoclopramide, erythromycin, cisapride, mosapride, tegaserod, prucalopride, itopride, and sumatriptan. A very promising compound is buspirone, a primarily 5HT1A agonist, that has been demonstrated to improve esophageal amplitude contractions post administration. In rare and severe symptomatic cases, esophagectomy may be considered.

Distal Esophageal Spasm and Jackhammer Esophagus

Distal esophageal spasm (DES) is the prototypical esophageal disorder in which patients present with chest pain and/or dysphagia. Because only the smooth muscle is affected with this disorder, the Chicago Classification renamed diffuse esophageal spasm as distal esophageal spasm. Patients with DES demonstrate normal IRP with at least 20% of swallows with DL <4.5 s. See Fig. 4.5b for high-resolution esophageal manometry image of distal esophageal spasm. The underlying pathophysiology for distal esophageal spasm is thought to be related to the disruption of inhibitory ganglionic neurons, thereby inducing premature, rapid, or simultaneous contractions in the muscularis propria. Some experts have hypothesized that DES is a precursor for achalasia. Though DES is considered a primary esophageal motor disorder, GERD and opiates have been associated with the manometric appearance of DES. The disorder is commonly described in patients presenting with chest pain. Classic esophagram findings include rosary beading and corkscrew esophagus.

Jackhammer esophagus is a hypercontractile esophageal disorder characterized by normal IRP and high amplitude contractions in the esophageal body (DCI >8000 mmHg·s·cm for ≥20% of swallows). Nutcracker esophagus, which was defined as DCI less than 8000 mmHg·s·cm, but greater than

5000 mmHg·s·cm for at least 10% of swallows, was removed from the latest version (3.0) of the Chicago Classification. See Fig. 4.5c for high-resolution esophageal manometry image of jackhammer esophagus. This is primarily because nutcracker esophagus was diagnosed in up to 5% of asymptomatic subjects based on the previous Chicago Classification version.

The pathophysiology behind Jackhammer esophagus is thought to be related to excess cholinergic stimulation of the circular muscle layer. Associated symptoms include chest pain, dysphagia, heartburn, and acid regurgitation. There has been some association between jackhammer esophagus, and eosinophilic esophagitis as well as evidence of progression to achalasia.

Both DES and jackhammer esophagus have been associated with esophagogastric junction (EGJ) outflow obstruction. Studies in animals and humans with EGJ outflow obstruction have shown esophageal hyperexcitability with high distal amplitude, multi-peaked contractions, and prolonged contraction duration. These findings have led to the speculation that hypercontractile esophageal disorders may progress to achalasia. Treatment of both DES and jackhammer esophagus include anti-reflux medications, pain modulators such as TCAs, SSRIs, trazodone, SNRIs, and smooth muscle relaxants such as nitrates, calcium channel blockers, and phosphodiesterase inhibitors. Opiates are also associated with these spastic disorders, and it is recommended to discontinue these medications if possible. Recently there have been small open-label trials in patients with jackhammer esophagus and DES treated with POEM with encouraging results.

EGJ Outflow Obstruction

EGJ outflow obstruction is a newly defined entity as per the Chicago Classification v3.0. It is defined as impaired EGJ relaxation at the time of swallowing and characterized by elevated median IRP (>15 mmHg) with normal or weak peristalsis. See Fig. 4.5d for high-resolution esophageal manometry image of EGJ outflow obstruction. It remains unclear as to what pathophysiology is behind this motor disorder. Patients with EGJ outflow obstruction commonly report dysphagia, typical or atypical symptoms of GERD. Patients with EGJ outflow obstruction should undergo upper endoscopy with mucosal biopsies to rule out subtle esophageal stricture, ring, infiltrative process, or eosinophilic esophagitis, as these entities can cause delay in esophageal bolus transit time and elevate the IRP value. If endoscopy is negative, it is recommended to proceed with barium swallow with a tablet or marshmallow or a timed barium esophagram. Some experts recommend endoscopic ultrasound in patients with EGJ outflow obstruction in order to rule out an esophageal wall lesion although the yield of such procedure is unknown. When evaluated by pH studies, only 17% of the patients with EGJ outflow obstruction demonstrate abnormal esophageal acid exposure.

Results from small trials comparing treatment of patients with EGJ outflow obstruction undergoing Heller myotomy, pneumatic dilation, or botulinum toxin A injection revealed no significant improvement of symptoms with any of the aforementioned therapeutic modalities. What is comforting though are some studies reporting spontaneous resolution of symptoms at 6 months without the need for treatment.

Minor Disorders of Peristalsis

There remains active debate regarding the clinical significance of the minor esophageal motor disorders. Ineffective esophageal motility (IEM) and fragmented peristalsis are two disorders that have been recently defined in the newest iteration of the Chicago Classification v3.0. IEM is defined by conventional manometry as mean amplitude contractions that are <30 mmHg, 3–8 cm above the LES. When using HREM, IEM is defined as at least 50% of the swallows are ineffective (either failed or weak) with DCI <450 mmHg·s·cm. Figure 4.5e depicts HREM of IEM. Multiple rapid swallows can also be used as a supplemental test to further evaluate patients with

IEM. Fragmented peristalsis is characterized by ≥50% fragmented contractions (large breaks >5 cm in the 20 mmHg isobaric contour) with DCI >450 mmHg·s·cm. Thus far, there are no studies that have determined the clinical significance of this disorder if any. IEM is considered the most common esophageal motor disorder with an estimated prevalence of 20–30%. The predominant symptom of IEM is dysphagia. There has been some association between IEM and GERD in the past, but further studies are needed to elucidate this relationship. The significance of esophageal minor motor disorders of peristalsis remains to be studied. However, due to the wide definition of IEM, even patients with severe motor abnormality fall under this category. For example, patients with 90% failed peristaltic swallows are considered as having IEM, although it is unlikely to be a minor motor disorder.

In patients warranting treatment, the first goal of therapy is to maximize acid suppression with double-dose PPI and possible H2 blocker at bedtime. If patients remain symptomatic, TLESR reducers can be used to help decrease symptomatic reflux events. Baclofen, a γ-aminobutyric acid (GABA) β-receptor agonist, acts to inhibit TLESRs and can be used up to three times a day. However, side effects such as fatigue and dizziness often limit its routine use in practice. Currently, there are no medications with consistent and effective effect on esophageal motility. Buspirone, a 5HT1A agonist, has demonstrated some promise in improving esophageal amplitude contractions and consequently dysphagia symptoms. Other potential therapeutic modalities and lifestyle modifications are mentioned under the absent contractibility section.

Secondary Esophageal Motility Disorders

Progressive Systemic Sclerosis

A number of conditions may affect the esophagus. Progressive systemic sclerosis (PSS) or scleroderma is the systemic disease most commonly associated with esophageal abnormalities in conjunction with its effect on skin, heart, lungs, and kidneys. Gastrointestinal tract involvement is seen in up to 90% of these patients, with the esophagus being the most commonly involved portion of the gastrointestinal tract. In up to 10% of patients, gastrointestinal tract manifestations may occur prior to the onset of other systemic manifestations.

In the gastrointestinal tract, PSS is manifested by injury to the smooth muscle layers. This includes atrophy of the muscle layer, collagen deposition, and sclerosis of arterioles. These changes lead to an irreversible injury to the esophageal smooth muscle resulting in progressive loss of esophageal peristalsis and eventually elimination of the LES. The following include typical changes in esophageal motility: (1) loss of peristalsis in the smooth muscle portion of the esophagus, (2) preservation of peristalsis in the skeletal muscle portion, and (3) very low or absent LES basal pressure. See Fig. 4.6 for

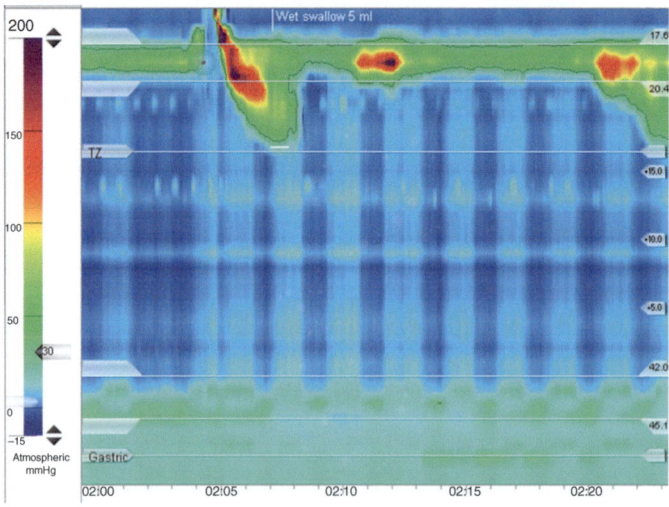

FIGURE 4.6 High-resolution esophageal manometry pattern of a patient with scleroderma. There is failed peristalsis on this swallow that involves only the smooth muscle part of the esophagus. Note preservation of peristalsis in the striated muscle part of the esophagus (S1)

high-resolution esophageal manometry image of scleroderma esophagus. The result of these changes is a disruption of the anti-reflux barrier and loss of the esophageal clearing mechanisms, which may lead to severe mucosal injury due to gastroesophageal reflux such as erosive esophagitis, esophageal stricture, and possible Barrett's metaplasia. In the era prior to the introduction of an effective acid-suppressive therapy, these patients were exposed to some acute complications of esophageal inflammation, including ulcer formation and life-threatening bleeding.

Other Esophageal Motility Disorders

Other connective tissue disorders may involve the esophagus. Mixed connective tissue (MCT) disease may cause a variety of manometric changes in the esophagus in both the smooth and skeletal muscle portions. Changes similar to those found in PSS may be present exposing patients to gastroesophageal reflux-related complications. A variety of manometric abnormalities may be noted in systemic lupus erythematous, mostly minor, although these changes do not commonly result in symptoms. Dysphagia is common in Sjogren's syndrome and may reflect a combination of the loss of saliva as a lubricant (xerostomia) and/or alterations in esophageal motility.

Alterations in esophageal motility may be seen in a wide variety of other conditions. Polymyositis affects principally the esophageal skeletal muscle and commonly result in transfer (oropharyngeal) dysphagia. Abnormal esophageal peristalsis can be seen in severe hypothyroidism and may result in dysphagia. Symptoms respond to thyroid replacement. Although manometric changes may be seen in hyperthyroidism, they are not commonly associated with symptoms. Similarly, a variety of manometric alterations may be seen in patients with diabetes mellitus, though most are not associated with symptoms.

References

1. Kahrilas PJ, Bredenoord AJ, Fox M, et al. The Chicago classification of esophageal motility disorders, v3.0. Neurogastroenterol Motil. 2015;27:160–74.
2. Boeckxstaens GE, Zaninotto G, Richter JE. Achalasia. Lancet. 2014;383:83–93.

Chapter 5
Esophageal Manifestations of Dermatological Conditions

Introduction

Patients with a personal or family history of dermatological conditions presenting with dysphagia should undergo evaluation for esophageal involvement of their dermatological condition.

Bullous Skin Disease with Esophageal Involvement

Epidermolysis bullosa (EB) is a genetic disorder characterized by blistering skin sores secondary to trauma and pressure to the skin [1]. Histopathologically it is defined by the separation of the dermis and the epidermis. The esophagus is affected in the dystrophic form of the disease, which is associated with mutations in the type VII collagen gene located on chromosome 3p21. Symptoms of dysphagia are more common in patients who inherit the recessive form of EB compared to those with the dominant inherited form (66% vs 20%, respectively). Early in life, patients experience esophageal bullae, scarring, and strictures, the latter of which occur more commonly in the proximal esophagus. Management of these patients includes treatment for GERD and esophageal candidiasis as well as nutritional therapy. For those requiring surgery, esophagectomy with colonic interposition may be offered.

Epidermolysis bullosa acquisita (EBA) is similar to EB but with milder skin symptoms and adult age of onset. It is also not genetically inherited. Associated conditions include amyloidosis, multiple myeloma, inflammatory bowel disease, and diabetes mellitus. Esophageal manifestations are rare but if present include proximal esophageal webs and strictures. On esophageal histopathology of EBA patients, IgG deposits are seen in a linear configuration in the basement membrane. Similar findings are seen on skin biopsy of these patients.

Pemphigus vulgaris (PV) is considered an autoimmune bullous skin disease affecting the stratified squamous epithelium. Diagnosis requires findings of IgG and C3 deposits of varying intensity under direct immunofluorescence and intercellular acantholysis, circulating antibodies bound to stratified squamous epithelium in active disease. PV affects the skin and mucous membranes in up to 90% of the patients. Although it is rare to have a significant esophageal involvement in PV despite symptoms of dysphagia and odynophagia, it is still advocated that all patients undergo endoscopic evaluation. Findings seen on upper endoscopy in PV patients include scattered red and white spots, longitudinal erythematous streaks, and esophagitis dissecans superficialis. The presence of the latter may be revealed when casts of the esophageal lining are vomited up. Endoscopy should be performed with caution given how fragile the mucosa can be in PV. Separation of the epidermis layers can be induced during endoscopy of these patients. The paraneoplastic form of PV, which is usually associated with lymphoreticular system malignancies, can also affect the esophagus. Treatment of esophageal lesions includes steroids and immunomodulators, including azathioprine and cyclophosphamide.

Cicatricial pemphigoid (CP) is an autoimmune bullous disease similar to PV but with a more benign course. It is most commonly seen in middle-age women and can affect ocular, oral, and other mucosal areas including the esophagus, larynx, and pharynx. The skin is only affected in 25% of patients, with esophageal involvement reported in approximately 4% of them manifested as proximal webs and strictures.

Stevens-Johnson syndrome is a severe form of erythema multiforme with acute eruptions of skin bullae and fever. Esophageal involvement presents with symptoms of dysphagia and gastrointestinal bleeding with findings of single or multiple erosions, likely related to erythema multiforme. Findings of denuded mucosa with white plaques represent esophageal necrosis. Recovery can be complicated with the formation of webs and strictures.

Herpes simplex virus (HSV) is associated with vesiculobullous skin disease usually localized to a given region on the body. In the disseminated form of HSV, the esophagus is the most common organ involved. Endoscopic findings are consistent with multiple ulcerations in the distal esophagus. Treatment of disseminated HSV involves a 14-day course of IV acyclovir.

Hailey-Hailey is an autosomal dominant inherited disease associated with blistering, crusting, and unpleasant smelling skin lesions in intertriginous areas and regions of skin trauma. Esophageal involvement is almost always an incidental finding, with patients rarely having symptoms. Treatment includes the use of topical and systemic steroids.

Darier's disease is similar to Hailey-Hailey but commonly affects the esophagus and occurs before age 20. Esophageal findings include keratotic papules and acanthosis similar to the skin lesions seen in these patients. Retinoids are used for treatment but are often poorly tolerated.

Hyperkeratotic Skin Disease with Esophageal Involvement

Lichen planus is a T-cell-mediated process that is considered an inflammatory process affecting the skin, mucous membranes, and nails. It appears on the skin as violaceous papules with a slight scale overlying. Esophageal involvement is rare and if present almost universally involves the oral mucosa by at least 2–5 years. Endoscopy reveals almost completely or fully denuded mucosa with white membranes on top and numerous proximal strictures. Biopsy of the esophagus will reveal dermal histiocytic infiltrate. There is a risk of developing squamous cell skin cancer, though there has been no association with malignancy risk when the esophagus is involved. Treatment includes inhaled or topical steroids.

Hyperkeratosis plantaris et palmaris (tylosis, Thost-Unna syndrome, Howel-Evans syndrome, diffuse palmoplantar keratoderma) is an autosomal dominant skin disease (chromosome 17q23), affecting the palms and soles. Skin findings include symmetric, regional, or diffuse thickening of the palms and soles with associated pruritus and deep fissures. Esophageal involvement includes endoscopic findings of papillomatosis (several small protrusions sometimes with spines secondary to acanthosis) and a 50% risk of squamous cell carcinoma (SCC) by age 45. Patients and family members should undergo regular screening of the esophagus for SCC. Esophagectomy is considered curative for endoscopic findings of advanced dysplasia.

Bazex syndrome (acrokeratosis neoplastica) is a paraneoplastic skin disease involving the hands and feet. It is associated with squamous cell carcinoma of the upper respiratory tract and esophagus. Early skin manifestations include psoriatic-like lesions on the finger digits and nail beds. The condition resolves with treatment of the underlying cancer.

Acanthosis nigricans (AN) can be idiopathic or associated with systemic conditions (e.g., systemic lupus erythematosus, dermatomyositis, scleroderma) and is characterized by numerous small velvety papillomatous plaques of the neck, arms, and axilla. Esophageal involvement is rare, but when present it can demonstrate squamous papilloma that has the potential to grow to large size and obstruct the lumen of the esophagus. AN is considered to be a paraneoplastic phenomenon and has been associated with gastric, pancreatic, colonic, and gallbladder adenocarcinoma, as well as hepatocellular cancer.

Collagen Vascular Disease

Scleroderma is a condition distinguished by its features of fibrosis and microvascular injury of affected organs. Approximately, 80% of patients develop esophageal involvement including refractory, complicated GERD secondary to abnormally low LES resting pressure and esophageal body dysmotility, specifically absent contractility (see Fig. 4.6). Mucosal findings of scleroderma esophagus include non-bleeding telangiectasia, esophageal inflammation (erosive esophagitis), and complications of GERD (peptic stricture and Barrett's esophagus). Patients with other connective tissue diseases such as Raynaud's phenomenon, mixed connective tissue disorder, and systemic lupus erythematosus may present with similar esophageal dysmotility patterns as scleroderma. Diagnosis is made by clinical history, physical examination, and laboratory tests with over 95% having a positive antinuclear antibody serum test and variable positivity to anti-topoisomerase or Scl-70. Management of these patients should include optimization of anti-reflux treatment to prevent its complications. Long-term results of surgical fundoplication have generally been disappointing and are not recommended. In very symptomatic patients, esophagectomy may be considered.

Dermatomyositis is an autoimmune disease that affects the skeletal muscle with the characteristic symptom of proximal limb weakness. Skin findings include the heliotrope rash, a violaceous rash affecting the upper eyelids, as well as scattered telangiectasias, eczematous and exfoliative dermatitis, and erythema. Overlap with other connective tissue diseases (i.e., scleroderma, systemic lupus erythematosus, and mixed connective tissue disease) is common. Esophageal skeletal muscle involvement (pharyngeal, cricopharyngeal, upper esophageal sphincter, and proximal esophagus) may present with symptoms of oropharyngeal dysphagia in up to 25% of patients. Abnormal esophageal manometry can be seen in up to 20% of patients.

Reference

1. Wise JL, Murray JA. Esophageal manifestations of dermatologic disease. Curr Gastroenterol Rep. 2002;4:205–12.

Chapter 6
Esophageal Malignancy

Introduction

Unlike most of the gastrointestinal tract, esophageal neoplasia is rarely benign. There has been an absolute increased incidence in esophageal carcinomas in the United States from 3.8 million diagnosed in 1973–1975 to 23.3 million in 2001. This increased incidence rate exceeds the rates of lung, breast, prostate, and melanoma cancers. It is estimated that in 2015, 17,000 new cases of esophageal cancer were diagnosed, representing 1% of all new cancer cases. In 2012, approximately 36,000 people in the United States were living with esophageal cancer. Despite increasing numbers of patients being diagnosed with esophageal cancer, the 5-year survival remains dismal (surveillance, epidemiology, and end results (SEER) program data). In some areas of the world, the incidence is much higher. Males are considered more at risk compared to females, with increasing risk with aging. Traditionally, African Americans and Asian patients are thought to have increased incidence of squamous cell carcinoma, while Caucasians are more likely to develop adenocarcinoma of the esophagus. In Western countries, there has been a decreasing incidence of squamous cell carcinoma of the esophagus in contrast to the marked increase in cases of esophageal adenocarcinoma. Incidence rates of esophageal adenocarcinoma have been exceeding 300% in both Caucasian men and women compared to prior decades. Diets that are high in red meat, fat, and processed food are associated with increased risk of both major types of esophageal malignancies.

Squamous Cell Carcinoma (SCC) of the Esophagus

When discussing this disease, it is critical to define the population at risk in the United States. Squamous cell carcinoma is a disease of African Americans, particularly males, and there is increased risk with aging. It is associated with alcohol (in particular whiskey and beer) and tobacco abuse (especially patients smoking more than 25 cigarettes per day) and have most notable deleterious effects when combined as they have synergistic carcinogenic effects. The reported incidence is approximately 2.6 per 100,000. In parts of China, this incidence in individuals without a history of tobacco and alcohol abuse is as high as 131.8 per 100,000. Other evidence of geographical clustering is reported in Central Asia, South Africa, and along the coast of South Carolina. Factors other than alcohol and tobacco abuse thought to contribute to an increased risk of squamous cell carcinoma of the esophagus include vitamin and mineral deficiencies, such as beta-carotene, B12, vitamin A, vitamin E, vitamin C, folic acid, molybdenum, zinc, and selenium, as well as the human papillomavirus (genotypes 16, 18, 33). Patients with the following conditions are noted to have an increased risk of SCC of the esophagus: long-standing achalasia, history of head and neck SCC, celiac sprue, atrophic gastritis, esophageal webs (i.e., Plummer-Vinson syndrome), history of consumption of a hot South American beverage (mate), history of prior gastrectomy, past history of caustic esophageal injury, and *tylosis palmaris et plantaris* (an autosomal dominant disease associated with hyperkeratosis of the palms and soles).

In clinical practice, patients with squamous cell carcinoma of the esophagus present with progressive solid food dysphagia [1]. Less commonly, patients may present with odynophagia, iron deficiency anemia, or hoarseness from injury to the recurrent laryngeal nerve. In some cases, complete esophageal obstruction may occur, leading to aspiration pneumonia. The mid esophagus is the most common site of SCC, followed by the distal esophagus and, much more uncommonly, the proximal esophagus.

Esophageal squamous cell carcinoma may metastasize to the nearby lymph nodes, liver, lung, and bone with symptoms attributable to disease extent. Under most circumstances, squamous cell cancer of the esophagus is not found at stage when cure is predictable. Five-year survival rates for squamous cell esophageal cancer are <10%. In areas of the world where the incidence is high enough to warrant screening, e.g., Linxian, China, a 5-year survival rate of 86% has been reported in patients found to have early SCC treated with esophagectomy [2].

Diagnosis

In the United States, the diagnosis is most often confirmed by endoscopic biopsy. The precursor lesions, squamous dysplasia, or squamous cell carcinoma in situ are rarely diagnosed because they tend to be asymptomatic. Endoscopy is commonly the first diagnostic test performed in patients with dysphagia. Small diameter scopes passed under direct vision can be used and thus obviate the need for a prior esophagram. See Fig. 6.1 for endoscopic appearance of squamous cell carcinoma. Following histologic confirmation of cancer, the tumor should be staged (depth of tumor penetration) and assessed for nodal involvement. See Fig. 6.2 for staging details. This is most appropriately done with a combination of computed tomography (CT) scan of the chest and endoscopic ultrasound (EUS). Evaluation of depth of invasion (T stage) into the wall and presence of regional lymph nodes (N stage) are most often accomplished with EUS. Accuracy of EUS for staging and assessment for locoregional lymph node involvement range from 70% to 80%. CT scan can accurately iden-

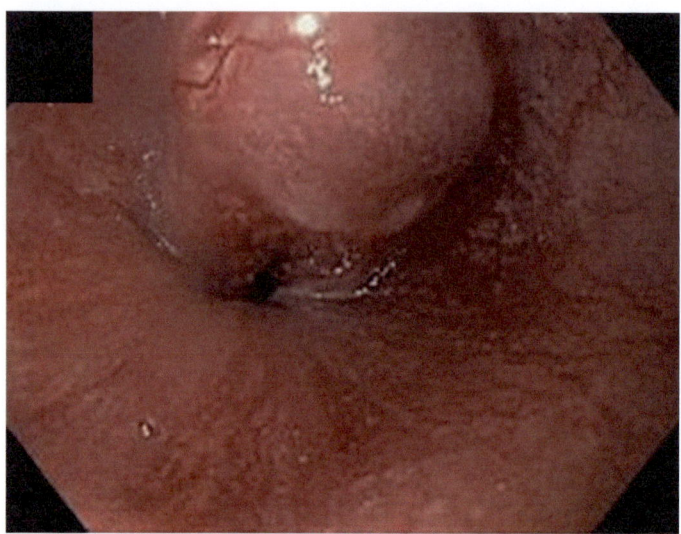

Figure 6.1 Endoscopic appearance of squamous cell carcinoma. A 2 cm tumor is seen in the lower esophagus

tify distant lymph node involvement and metastatic disease. Emerging data also posits a role for 18F-fluoro-2-deoxy-D-glucose positron emission tomography (FDG-PET) for similar assessment of distant lymph nodes or metastatic disease as CT, perhaps with even greater accuracy.

Treatment

In patients presenting with squamous cell carcinoma of the esophagus, surgery represents the best chance for long-term, disease-free survival. However, most patients with this disease usually present late, in which time surgical cure is not possible. Multiple studies have been published evaluating the tumor response to multimodality therapy. This includes combination of chemotherapy, radiotherapy, and potentially surgical intervention when the tumor is downstaged. Endoscopic therapies are most commonly used in recent

Squamous Cell Carcinoma (SCC) of the Esophagus

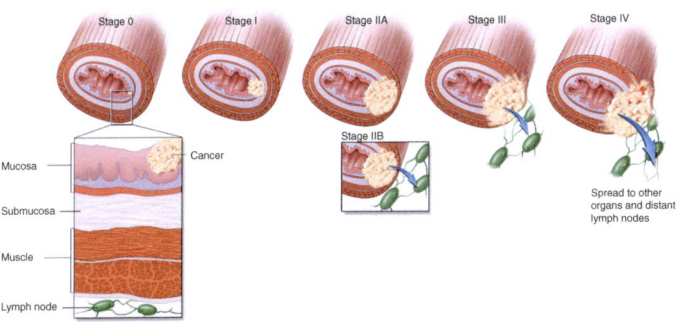

FIGURE 6.2 Simplified staging of esophageal carcinoma. Stages 0 through IV are used to classify carcinoma characterized by different degrees of tumor invasion, lymph node involvement, and metastasis. Stage 0 are intramucosal tumors that do not invade the lamina propria. Stage I tumors invade the lamina propria without lymph node or distant involvement. Stage II tumors extend to the muscle layer either without (IIA) or with (IIB) lymph node involvement. Stage III tumors invade through the muscular layer and involve lymph nodes or other adjacent structures. Stage IV tumors spread to distant organs or lymph nodes. (With permission from Bhaijee, F. Staging of esophageal carcinoma. PathologyOutlines.com website. http://www.pathologyoutlines.com/topic/esophagusstaging.html. Accessed March 5th, 2018)

years for inoperable cases. Treatment for patients with esophageal cancer should be individualized. The gastroenterologist's involvement with squamous cell carcinoma often includes palliation for progressive dysphagia or tracheoesophageal fistula by repeated dilations, placement of percutaneous gastrostomy, control of bleeding, or placement of esophageal stent. Early stage squamous cell carcinoma of the esophagus could be removed by an expert endoscopist using the endoscopic mucosal resection (EMR) technique. In addition to stent placement, other palliative therapies are available, and they include bougienage (dilation), laser, argon beam coagulation, photodynamic therapy, endoscopic ethanol injection, external beam radiotherapy, intraluminal brachytherapy, palliative resection, and bypass surgeries.

Adenocarcinoma of the Esophagus

Over the past 50 years, there has been a significant increase in the incidence of adenocarcinoma of the esophagus in Westernized societies. Presently 50–80% of all esophageal cancers in the United States are adenocarcinoma of the esophagus.

Furthermore, adenocarcinoma of the esophagus is one of the fastest rising cancers in the United States and is the second most common esophageal cancer in the world. Before 1978, based on a surgical series, esophageal adenocarcinoma was considered uncommon. It was only after 1994 that the prevalence of esophageal adenocarcinoma surpassed that of squamous cell carcinoma in the United States. There has been over 400% and 300% increase in incidence of esophageal adenocarcinoma in both Caucasian men and women, respectively, since 1970 with an incidence rate estimated to be 5.3 per 100,000 persons. Patients with both esophageal squamous cell carcinoma and esophageal adenocarcinoma early in their disease often do not have symptoms. However, as the disease progresses, patients present to health-care providers with symptoms of progressive dysphagia to both solids and liquids and weight loss. Late diagnosis of these cancers is often made because patients modify their diets over time due to dysphagia symptoms. Rarely, patients will present with odynophagia, and usually it indicates the presences of ulceration of the malignancy or superimposed candida infection. In addition, patients may present with recurrent pneumonias and pleural effusions indicative of esophageal respiratory fistula that may have formed due to tumor invasion into adjacent pulmonary structures. Hoarseness may also occur due to compression of the recurrent laryngeal nerve from tumor burden or lymphadenopathy. Adenocarcinoma of the esophagus almost exclusively arises from Barrett's esophagus, which has been directly linked to gastroesophageal reflux disease (GERD). Other additional risk factors that have been associated with esophageal adenocarcinoma include higher socioeconomic

Adenocarcinoma of the Esophagus

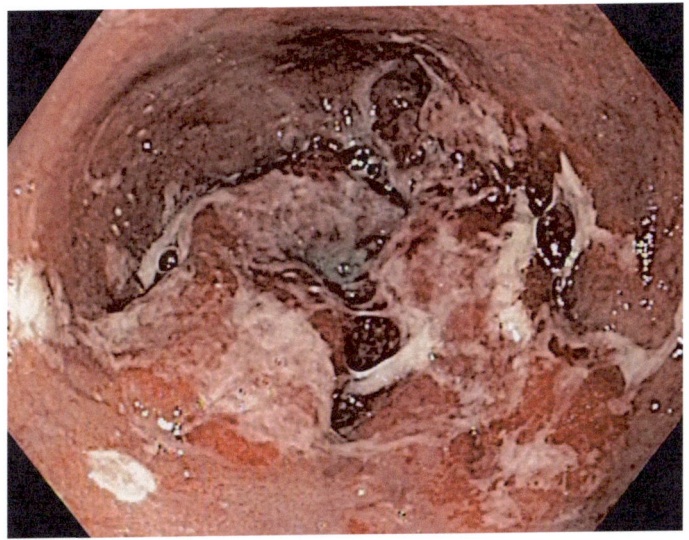

FIGURE 6.3 Endoscopic appearance of esophageal adenocarcinoma. Patient presented with progressive dysphagia symptoms and weight loss with findings of almost completely obstructive esophageal adenocarcinoma in the distal esophagus

status, obesity, tobacco smoking, Caucasian race, and male sex. Both *H. pylori* infection and NSAIDs have been suggested to be protective against esophageal adenocarcinoma. See Fig. 6.3 for endoscopic appearance of esophageal adenocarcinoma.

Diagnosis

Much like squamous cell carcinoma of the esophagus, adenocarcinoma of the esophagus is diagnosed by esophageal mucosal biopsies performed at the time of upper endoscopy. Water-soluble radiographic contrast esophagram can be used to evaluate for suspected complications related to esophageal adenocarcinoma such as tracheoesophageal fistulas. The yield of endoscopic diagnosis can be increased with adjunctive tools such as multiple biopsies; endoscopic imaging techniques such as chromoendoscopy, narrow-band imaging, autofluorescence imaging, and confocal endomicroscopy. These techniques can help in identifying areas of dysplasia and malignancy during endoscopy. Once confirmed, esophageal adenocarcinoma should be further staged with EUS to assess depth of invasion, chest CT, and PET scanning to assess for metastatic disease. Treatment of esophageal adenocarcinoma is further discussed under "Barrett's esophagus."

Barrett's Esophagus (BE)

According to the guidelines for the diagnosis, surveillance, and therapy for Barrett's esophagus (BE) published by the American College of Gastroenterology, Barrett's esophagus is defined as a change in the esophageal epithelium of any length that can be recognized at endoscopy and is confirmed to have intestinal metaplasia by biopsy from the tubular esophagus. Both Barrett's esophagus and esophageal adenocarcinoma are much less common in non-Caucasian populations. It is considered to be an acquired condition associated with GERD. Of those undergoing endoscopy for any reason, 1–2% may have Barrett's esophagus, while in those undergoing endoscopy for GERD-related symptoms, between 6% and 10% of patients harbor Barrett's esophagus. Risk factors associated with the development of BE include long-standing GERD (≥ 5 years), Caucasian ethnicity, obesity, tobacco use, family history of esophageal adenocarcinoma or BE, and hiatal hernia. Patients symptomatic with GERD are more likely to have long segment BE (LSBE) compared to short segment BE (SSBE). The incidence of Barrett's esophagus is clearly underestimated. It is estimated that up to 50% of patients with Barrett's esophagus do not have symptoms of GERD, and thus even an aggressive screening program in patients with chronic heartburn complaints will miss a substantial number of cases. Given these challenges in identifying patients at risk for esophageal adenocarcinoma, techniques for screening have been developed to help diagnose BE with acceptable sensitivity and specificity and decreased cost. These techniques include unsedated transnasal endoscopy (uTNE) (sensitivity 98%, specificity 100%) and cytosponge with protein marker trefoil factor 3 (sensitivity 73%, specificity 94%).

The actual incidence of adenocarcinoma in patients with Barrett's esophagus is low. Although the risk of developing adenocarcinoma is 30–125 times that of the non-Barrett's patients, non-dysplastic BE, low-grade dysplasia, and high-grade dysplasia have adenocarcinoma incidence rates of 0.12–0.40% per year, 1% per year, and 5% per year, respectively. Factors implicated as being protective against the development of esophageal adenocarcinoma include a diet high in fruits and vegetables, NSAIDs, and *Helicobacter pylori* infection.

Many authors divide Barrett's esophagus into short segment (SSBE) and long segment (LSBE). This distinction is based on the length of the metaplastic epithelium (SBE <3 cm, LSBE ≥3 cm). Another method used to describe the extent of Barrett's mucosa is the prague circumference (C) and maximum (M) criteria. The length of Barrett's esophagus is divided to the circumferential part of the columnar-like epithelium (if present), and the part that is only composed from metaplastic tongues. It is more common to find dysplasia in patients with LSBE, and there is a correlation between the length of Barrett's epithelium and the risk of developing dysplasia. Some preliminary data suggest that the cancer risk is also increased in patients with SSBE as compared to subject without Barrett's esophagus. Adenocarcinoma in the setting of Barrett's esophagus involves changes at the cellular level, which result in histological and then ultimately morphological changes. The genetic alterations described in the neoplastic progression of Barrett's esophagus include expression of oncogenes (e.g., cyclin D1 and K-ras), growth factors and receptors (TGF-α, EGF receptor), and inactivation of tumor suppressor genes such as TP53 and p16. As the process proceeds, often in association with the development of dysplasia, aneuploid populations of DNA may be found in the nucleus of cells in the metaplastic epithelium. It is the emergence of dysplasia that determines the population at highest risk for the subsequent development of adenocarcinoma.

Given the risk of adenocarcinoma development, surveillance of patients with Barrett's esophagus is recommended. Lack of large-scale studies, which provide the base for surveillance recommendations, led to a variety of guidelines which are based on presumed risk. Because inflammation can mimic the cellular/nuclear changes often seen with dysplasia, all patients with Barrett's esophagus should be placed on adequate acid suppression therapy, i.e., proton pump inhibitors prior to endoscopy and biopsy. Even if anti-reflux surgery has been performed, a surveillance program is still warranted.

Under most circumstances, patients with Barrett's esophagus without dysphagia should have an endoscopic surveillance within 1 year of diagnosis and if unremarkable the next after 3 years and afterwards at 5-year intervals. Multiple biopsies are taken every 2 cm at 4 quadrants in patients without dysplasia and every 1 cm intervals in those with prior dysplasia. It is agreeable today that columnar tongues less than 1 cm in length should not be biopsied for the presence of intestinal metaplasia. Even with such a careful exam, some series report up to 13% of resected esophagi to harbor invasive cancer in patients diagnosed with high-grade dysplasia. Biopsies should be reviewed by a pathologist familiar with Barrett's metaplasia. If dysplasia of any degree is found, these biopsies should be forwarded to another pathologist specializing in Barrett's histopathology given the high interobserver variability in agreement on diagnosis (interobserver agreement on low-grade dysplasia is less than 50% vs approximately 85% for high-grade dysplasia).

Dysplasia is defined as cytological and architectural abnormalities on histopathology favoring unchecked cell growth. It is typically categorized as low-grade dysplasia (LGD), high-grade dysplasia (HGD), or indefinite for dysplasia. High-grade dysplasia is considered to have more potential for carcinogenesis with histological findings that suggest more severe genetic damage. In some series, a significant number of BE patients with HGD will already have intramucosal adenocarcinoma. In one prospective evaluation of a group of patients with HGD, less than 20% developed adenocarcinoma during a 17-year follow-up. Given the age of this population with a host of comorbid conditions, most are likely to die from causes other than adenocarcinoma of the esophagus.

Patients with confirmed HGD have three management options that include esophagectomy, mucosal ablation, or frequent surveillance. Esophagectomy is the only way to guarantee that a patient will not develop adenocarcinoma of the esophagus over time. Surveillance only for HGD is not commonly offered anymore primarily because of the intensity of follow-ups and the availability of safe and efficacious alternative options. However, in those who do not wish to undergo surgical or endoscopic treatment or who are not candidates for these procedures, frequent surveillance is commonly offered. Endoscopic treatment for HGD includes endoscopic mucosal resection (EMR) and ablative therapy.

EMR is used in patients with mucosal irregularity (i.e., nodules, ulceration, irregular mucosal contour) in BE which are confirmed to harbor high-grade dysplasia and/or adenocarcinoma limited to the mucosa (T1a lesions). This modality uses a diathermic snare or endoscopic knife to resect Barrett's epithelium down to the submucosa, which can subsequently be submitted for pathological evaluation of extent and adequacy of resection.

Ablative techniques employed in the treatment of LGD, HGD, and adenocarcinoma limited to the mucosa include photodynamic therapy, radiofrequency ablation, cryoablation, and argon plasma coagulation. Complete endoscopic eradication of Barrett's esophagus is not currently recommended in patients with non-dysplastic Barrett's esophagus, due to the low risk of neoplastic progression.

All patients with Barrett's esophagus, regardless of the chosen treatment modality, should receive a PPI to control GERD-related symptoms and possible delay neoplastic progression. Unfortunately, most patients with adenocarcinoma of the esophagus will present at a stage when curative surgery is not often an option. As with squamous cell carcinoma of the esophagus, physicians are faced with issues of staging and initiating an aggressive chemotherapy program and/or radiotherapy as a mean of downstaging the cancer. In many situations, the gastroenterologist will again serve as the person responsible for providing palliative therapy in the setting of advanced disease.

Other Esophageal Tumors

Other malignant tumors of the esophagus include verrucous carcinoma, carcinosarcoma, small-cell carcinoma, and malignant melanoma of the esophagus. Verrucous carcinoma and carcinosarcoma are variants of squamous cell carcinoma, with the former described as being a warty-appearing lesion with acanthosis, hyperkeratosis, and a small number of neoplastic cells on histology. On the other hand, carcinosarcoma (also known as spindle cell carcinoma, polypoid carcinoma, and pseudosarcoma) is defined by a polypoid appearance on endoscopy and symptoms of dysphagia or epigastric pain. Histologically these tumors demonstrate spindle cells and often present in an advanced stage with metastasis to regional lymph nodes at the time of diagnosis. Small-cell carcinoma accounts for very few esophageal tumors and just like its pulmonary counterpart, it is an aggressive tumor with overall poor prognosis. The tumor presents in the mid- to lower esophagus in 30–50% of the time, respectively, with over 50% of patients demonstrate metastatic disease at diagnosis. Men more commonly are afflicted with this type of cancer compared to women. Associated risk factors include tobacco and alcohol use. Malignant melanoma of the esophagus is also often metastatic on presentation with histological findings of melanocytes in the basal epithelium of the esophagus. Men are more commonly affected than women. Dysphagia symptoms are often late in the disease due to the soft pliable nature of this tumor which is commonly located in mid- to distal regions of the esophagus. Endoscopically it appears as a non-ulcerated, pigmented tumor with color being determined by the concentration of melanin.

Benign epithelial tumors of the esophagus include squamous papilloma, adenoma, and inflammatory fibroid polyp. squamous papilloma is most often encountered as an incidental finding on endoscopy and are characterized as a single lesion that is exophytic in appearance in the distal esophagus (see Fig. 6.4 for endoscopic appearance of squamous papilloma). They account for less than 1% of the esophageal tumors and have theoretical association with an underlying inflammatory condition such as GERD or the human papillomavirus (HPV). Due to their generally small size, most can be resected at the time of endoscopy. Squamous papilloma has low rate of recurrence and malignant potential. Certain

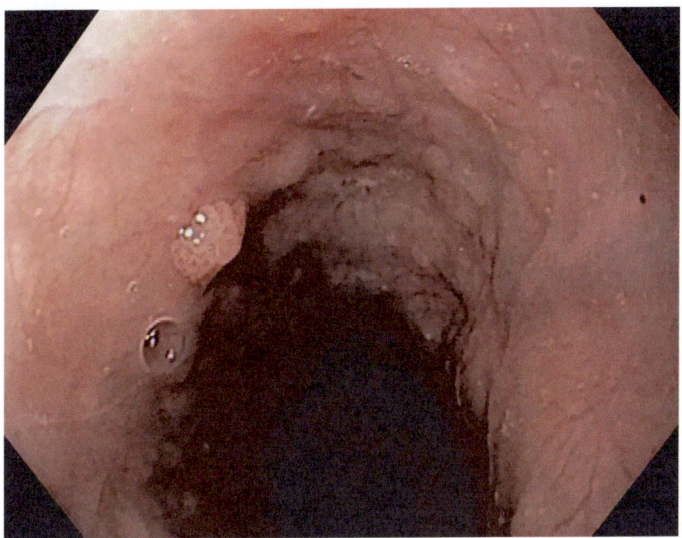

FIGURE 6.4 Endoscopic appearance of squamous papilloma. Patient undergoing routine endoscopy for GERD symptoms with incidental finding of a squamous papilloma in the proximal esophagus

genotypes of HPV have been shown to be associated with squamous papilloma and increased malignant potential.

Lymphomas of the esophagus, of either the Hodgkin's or non-Hodgkin's type, comprise less than 1% of all esophageal malignancies and present endoscopically as submucosal nodules, ulcerations, mass, or polypoid-like lesions. Gastrointestinal stromal tumors (GISTs) are found in 1–3% of the time in the esophagus and are seen in the distal esophagus as subepithelial solitary masses on endoscopy. Esophageal GISTs that are greater than 2 cm in size or with greater than 5 mitosis per high-power field are associated with greater malignant potential. The two most common cancers to metastasize to the esophagus are breast and melanoma, which oftentimes are found incidentally by externally compressing the esophagus. Leiomyomas are the most common benign nonepithelial esophageal tumor, affecting men twice as often as women. These lesions are often present as a single or multiple submucosal mass with normal overlying esophageal mucosa. An EUS exam helps to diagnose these lesions, which arise from the muscularis propria. Granular cell tumors are found in the esophagus 33% of the time and present as solitary yellowish tumor with cells containing eosinophilic-rich cytoplasm, which are periodic Schiff-positive and diastase-resistant. Pedunculated polyps in the esophagus are most commonly identified as either (1) fibrovascular polyps seen in the proximal esophagus composed of stroma, adipose cells and blood vessels, or (2) hamartomas, which often contain several different types of tissue (e.g., cartilage, adipose, skeletal muscle, and bone). Lastly, both esophageal hemangiomas, vascular-appearing submucosal nodules, and lipomas, yellowish raised nodules in the proximal esophagus, are rare findings of the esophagus.

References

1. Ohashi S, Miyamoto S, Kikuchi O, et al. Recent advances from basic and clinical studies of esophageal squamous cell carcinoma. Gastroenterology. 2015;149:1700–15.
2. Rustgi AK, El-Serag HB. Esophageal carcinoma. N Engl J Med. 2014;371:2499–509.

Chapter 7
Rings and Webs

Introduction

Nosology is critical when discussing rings and webs. An esophageal ring is defined as a distal esophageal structure which is mostly composed of mucosa. Muscular rings may also occur in the esophagus, although are less common. Esophageal webs refer to thin horizontal membranes stratified squamous epithelium that are most commonly located in the cervical (proximal) and mid esophagus.

Rings

Commonly, rings only partially occlude the esophageal lumen. Barium esophagram identifies esophageal rings and classify them based on their location in the esophagus. An A ring is a muscular ring occurring 2 cm proximal to the squamocolumnar junction at the proximal margin of the LES. B ring is located at the esophagogastric junction and is covered on one side by squamous mucosa and on the other side by columnar mucosa. The presence of symptoms is dictated by the ring diameter. Schatzki's ring is a type of B ring and is oftentimes between 12.5 and 20 mm in diameter.

Lower esophageal ring (Schatzki's ring) is thought to be the most common cause of dysphagia (see Fig. 7.1). The history

64 Chapter 7. Rings and Webs

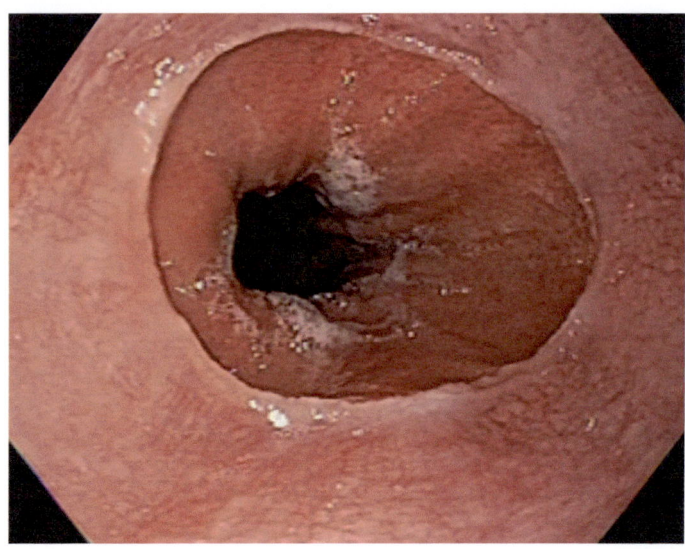

FIGURE 7.1 Endoscopic appearance of Schatzki's ring. Patient presented to endoscopy with symptoms of intermittent solid food dysphagia over the last 1–2 years with findings of a Schatzki's ring in the distal esophagus

of patient's complaints is characteristic. The patient is typically older than age 40 (although younger patients may be affected as well). The patient notices intermittent, early meal, and solid food dysphagia. The dysphagia is usually transient, and if the bolus passes, the remainder of the meal can be consumed. Patients may go for many weeks without symptoms. Importantly, symptoms are not progressive, and constitutional symptoms such as weight loss are absent. Occasionally these patients may require evaluation for food impaction.

Rings are diagnosed either radiographically or endoscopically. Rings may show varying degrees of narrowing. Rings with a luminal diameter of 13 mm or greater are much more likely to be asymptomatic, although other factors including bolus size and effectiveness of esophageal peristalsis are thought to contribute to intermittent episodes of dysphagia. Esophageal rings have been associated with eosinophilic esophagitis and should be considered in the differential diagnosis in patients with recurrent esophageal rings. The pathogenesis of rings is not well established. Current research has focused on the likely contribution of acidic reflux to the formation of these rings. There is a growing body of literature suggesting that many of the patients respond to acid-suppressive therapy with proton pump inhibitors, both in terms of decreased size of the rings and reduced symptoms. In some patients, esophageal bougienage or more aggressive endoscopic manipulation (four quadrant needle knife incision) may be required.

Esophageal webs refer to thin horizontal membranes stratified squamous epithelium that are most commonly located in the cervical (proximal) and mid esophagus. Cervical esophageal webs are typically diaphragmatic-like structures found in the immediate post-cricoid area. They are found in up to 5% of asymptomatic patients as incidental findings on imaging or endoscopy. They may be easily missed with by the aforementioned diagnostic modalities if care is not taken to carefully examine this area of the esophagus. The pathogenesis of cervical webs is unknown. Pathologically, they are composed of normal squamous tissue over connective tissue. This typical histology separated these cervical webs from changes in the proximal esophagus that are consistent with dermatological diseases, e.g., epidermolysis bullosa, pemphigoid, and chronic graft-versus-host disease.

Symptomatic patients are more likely to be female. Typically, the symptom complex is intermittent solid food dysphagia. When associated with iron deficiency anemia, this is referred to as Paterson-Kelly or Plummer-Vinson syndrome, which has been associated with an increased risk of development of squamous cell carcinoma of the pharynx and esophagus. Management of a typical cervical web is usually quite simple. Iron supplement in patients with iron deficiency often results in resolution of dysphagia and disappearance of the webs. Most webs can be disrupted during the routine performance of endoscopy, demonstrating how thin and fragile these structures often are. In some patients, esophageal bougienage may be required.

Mid-esophageal webs are associated with other systemic diseases such as graft-versus-host. Although typically found in the proximal esophagus, dermatologic diseases such as epidermolysis bullosa and pemphigoid may produce mid-esophageal webs. Other unusual cases include psoriasis and Steven-Johnson's syndrome.

In an otherwise normal population, an entity characterized by multiple esophageal webs has been described. These patients are, typically young adults, present with intermittent solid food dysphagia and/or food impaction. Endoscopically, multiple webs can be visualized in the upper, mid, and lower esophagus, in two adjacent areas or throughout the whole esophagus. Barium esophagram is not sensitive enough for the detection of multiple esophageal webs, as normal esophagram has been reported in published series. Furthermore, the radiographic abnormalities were often subtle and can simulate tertiary contractions. Endoscopy is the most accurate method of diagnosis. This entity has been recognized with increasing frequency. It has been given different names including feline esophagus, congenital funnel-shaped esophagus, and multiple esophageal webs. The etiology is unknown. Pathologically, an intense inflammatory infiltrate with eosinophils has been described. The critical issue with this entity is to recognize the need to dilate these rings with caution. In a small number of published series, the risk of perforation appears to be not uncommon.

Suggested Reading

1. Gasiorowska A, Fass R. Current approach to dysphagia. Gastroenterol Hepatol. 2009;5:269–79.

Chapter 8
Esophageal Diverticula

Introduction

Diverticula of the esophagus represent outpouchings of the esophagus and are considered pseudodiverticula (lacking muscular portions of the esophageal wall). In the past, diverticula have been classified as pulsion or traction. However, studies have determined that most diverticula (Zenker, midesophageal, and epiphrenic) represent the long-term outcome of altered esophageal motility. If required, treatment may be directed at the diverticulum itself and/or the associated motility abnormality.

Zenker's Diverticulum

Zenker's diverticulum actually represents a hypopharyngeal diverticulum. The diverticulum commonly presents with dysphagia, regurgitation, and may also present difficulties in passing the endoscope. Zenker's diverticulum is a pseudodiverticulum formed as the hypopharyngeal mucosa protrudes posteriorly and to the left between the thyropharyngeal and cricopharyngeal fibers of the inferior pharyngeal constrictor muscle. While it has been proposed that abnormal relaxation or poor compliance of the upper esophageal sphincter (UES) may result in increase in intra-pharyngeal pressure and thus the formation of Zenker's diverticulum, it has been very difficult to prove by either manometric or radiographic studies. Zenker's diverticulum is an acquired lesion that is found most commonly in men (with 2:1 prevalence of men vs women) during their seventh or 8th decade of life. Zenker's diverticulum may be found incidentally at the time of an esophagram performed for other reasons, with an estimated prevalence of 0.1–0.01%. Symptoms attributed to these diverticula include regurgitation, dysphagia, cough with or without aspiration pneumonia, weight loss, or a mass in the neck following eating (typically on the left side of the neck). See Fig. 8.1 for barium esophagram finding of Zenker's diverticulum [1]. If endoscopy is attempted, care must be exercised since the presence of a large Zenker's diverticulum forced the actual esophageal lumen anteriorly. If passed blinding, the scope will preferentially enter the diverticulum, and there is an increased risk of perforation. Some authors have recommended having the patient swallow a string, which can be followed by the endoscopist into the tubular esophagus. Symptomatic diverticula typically require surgical or endoscopic treatment. Treatment options include (1) excision of the diverticulum, (2) cricopharyngeal myotomy, (3) diverticulopexy (lifting the diverticulum), or (4) rigid endoscopic resection of the wall between the diverticulum and the esophagus. The latter procedure has been used for patients who are symptomatic yet poor surgical risks. Considerations must be given to an increased risk of aspiration in patients with gastroesophageal reflux with Zenker's diverticulum, if a myotomy is performed.

Mid-esophageal Diverticula

Mid-esophageal diverticula are typically found at the level of the bifurcation of the trachea (T4-T5). These diverticula are found more often on the right than on the left of the

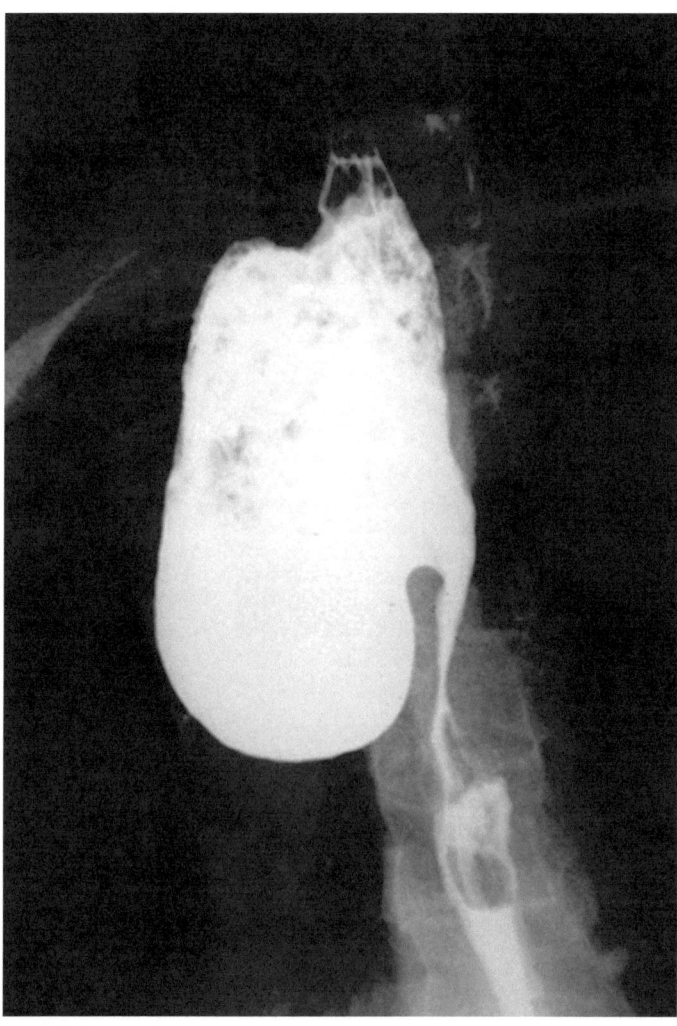

FIGURE 8.1 Barium esophagram appearance of Zenker's diverticulum. Barium esophagram was obtained prior to surgery with findings of a large Zenker's diverticulum extending deep into the chest. (With permission from Zhang et al. [1])

esophagus. See Fig. 8.2 for endoscopic appearance of mid-esophageal diverticula. In some of the original studies, these diverticula were found in association with mediastinal lymph nodes, which were currently or had been infected with tuberculosis. This led to the term traction diverticula, suggesting that the inflammatory reaction pulled the esophageal wall and created the diverticula. Traction diverticula have been associated with infection (tuberculosis, histoplasmosis), fibrosis, or an external neoplastic process. In contrast, pulsion diverticula are associated with altered esophageal motility, with symptoms more likely related to the esophageal dysmotility rather than the diverticulum. Most commonly, they are found incidentally at the time of endoscopy or radiographic studies. No therapy is required except in the very unusual situation where symptoms are

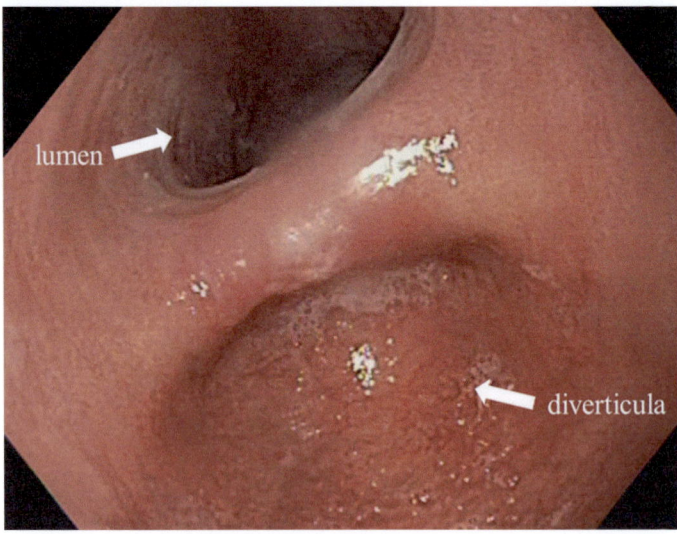

FIGURE 8.2 Endoscopic appearance of a mid-esophageal diverticula. Patient presented with intermittent symptoms of dysphagia and GERD for several years prior to endoscopy. There is moderate size mid-esophageal diverticulum noted at the time of endoscopy

thought to be related to the diverticulum. Surgery can be considered in patients with ongoing symptoms of dysphagia, aspiration, or when the size of the diverticulum exceeds 5 cm.

Epiphrenic Diverticula

Epiphrenic diverticula occur in the distal esophagus, typically 4–8 cm above the cardia. They may be single or multiple and are usually found on the right side of the esophagus. See Fig. 8.3 for the endoscopic appearance of epiphrenic diverticula. This form of diverticula has provided the most convincing information to support altered motility as an etiology. Several reports suggest that as many as 80% of the patients have an established motility disorder (achalasia, diffuse esophageal spasm, or hypertensive LES). They have also been found following bariatric surgery, in particular post-

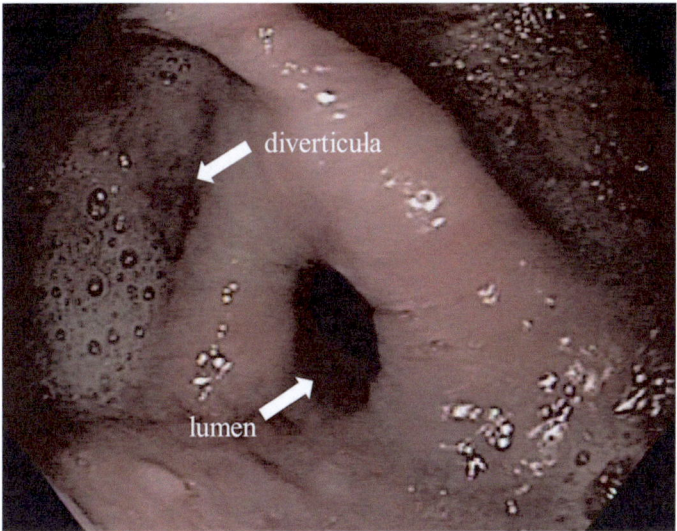

FIGURE 8.3 Endoscopic appearance of an epiphrenic diverticula. Patient presented with intermittent symptoms of dysphagia

gastric banding surgeries. They are commonly seen in the sixth decade of life, with a male predominance. Most patients are asymptomatic, although dysphagia, regurgitation, and chest pain may occur. Squamous cell carcinoma of the esophagus has been reported in association with epiphrenic diverticula.

Determining if the patient's symptoms are related to the diverticulum or the underlying motility disorder may be difficult. If treatment is necessary, a careful preoperative evaluation including endoscopy and manometry is required. If an associated motility disorder is present, it must be addressed at the time of surgery. Removal of the diverticulum alone is associated with increased morbidity and mortality, and these diverticula will likely recur.

Miscellaneous Diverticula

Other uncommon types of esophageal diverticula may be encountered. Esophageal intramural pseudodiverticulosis is an entity in which multiple small outpouchings of the esophageal mucosa are seen endoscopically or radiographically. They represent dilated excretory ducts of deep esophageal mucous glands. This entity typically presents with stricture formation. Associations with Candida infection, caustic ingestion, esophageal cancer, eosinophilic esophagitis, and GERD have been reported. See Fig. 8.4 for a barium esophagram and endoscopic appearance of esophageal intramural pseudodiverticulosis [2]. Congenital diverticula have been reported as a consequence of incomplete esophageal duplication.

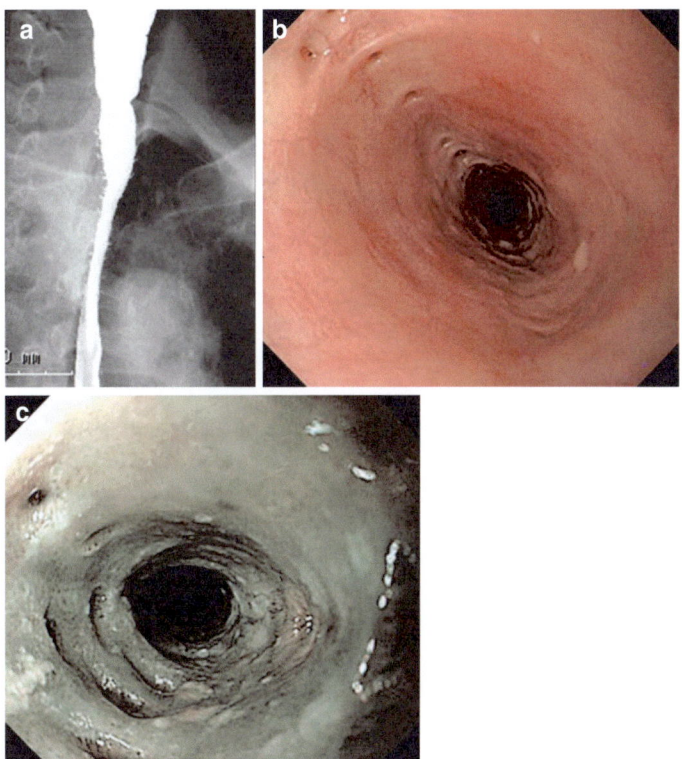

FIGURE 8.4 Barium esophagram and endoscopic appearance of esophageal intraluminal pseudodiverticulosis. Barium esophagram (**a**) showed a stricture of the thoracic esophagus with multiple small flank- or collar-button-shaped outpouchings in the cervical esophagus. Esophagoscopy showed multiple small orifices at the cervical esophagus (**b**). With narrowband imaging (NBI) pseudodiverticula were revealed more clearly as brown-colored holes than white light imaging. Magnifying endoscopy with NBI showed brownish areas in the mucosal orifices and homogeneously dilated and regularly arranged microvessels around the orifices (**c**). (With permission from Yamamoto et al. [2])

References

1. Zhang X, Cheng S, Xu Y, et al. Treatment of giant pharyngoesophageal diverticulum by video-assisted thoracoscopy. Ann Thorac Surg. 2014;97:2184–6.
2. Yamamoto S, Tsutsui S, Hayashi N. Esophageal intramural pseudodiverticulosis: a rare cause of esophageal stricture. Clin Gastroenterol Hepatol. 2010;8:A28.

Chapter 9
Vascular Abnormalities of the Esophagus

Dysphagia Lusoria

Abnormalities of the aortic arch, specifically the right aortic arch with an aberrant right subclavian artery, can press upon the trachea and esophagus causing partial or complete compression and collapse. Patients with this type of compression of the esophagus with symptoms of dysphagia are described as having dysphagia lusoria. On upper endoscopy, the pulsating aberrant right subclavian artery appears as an extrinsic compression on the esophagus along the posterior wall, with no abnormal mucosal findings. Prevalence of an aberrant right subclavian artery ranges from 0.5% to 1.8% of the general population. Other etiologies of extrinsic compression of the esophagus that may cause symptoms of dysphagia include mediastinal masses (e.g., germ cell tumor, lymphoma, and thyroid carcinoma), aortic arch aneurysm, and vertebral spurs. Diagnostic modalities used to visualize dysphagia lusoria include chest X-ray, CT scan, MRI, multidetector computed tomography angiography, and upper endoscopy [1]. The majority of causes of dysphagia lusoria are discovered incidentally on studies performed for other reasons.

Reference

1. Alper F, Akgun M, Kantarci M, et al. Demonstration of vascular abnormalities compressing esophagus by MDCT: special focus on dysphagia lusoria. Eur J Radiol. 2006;59:82–7.

Chapter 10
Foreign Bodies

Introduction

Foreign bodies represent a common problem for the clinical gastroenterologist. Management principles are based on the nature of the ingested material and its location in the gastrointestinal tract. The esophagus is one of the locations where intervention is often required. The nature of the ingested material is often a function of the age of the population, along with cultural variation in diet and the unique populations that may be encountered (e.g., patients with mental illness and prisoners). Underlying alterations in the lumen of the esophagus also play an important role in the risk of a swallowed object becoming lodged.

Pediatric Population

In the pediatric population, the swallowed objects may be relatively innocuous, while others can result in morbidity and mortality (e.g., button batteries). Coins are frequently swallowed by children. Additionally, the ethnic background may expose children to specific foreign bodies. For example, traditional Chinese food often contains multiple small bones, which may be lodged within the esophagus.

Special Circumstances

Special circumstances include patients with mental illness who may ingest any type of material. Prisoners will often ingest foreign bodies, many with the intent to induce perforation and the need for surgery. In the elderly, loose-fitting dentures pose a specific risk not likely to be encountered elsewhere.

Nosology of Foreign Bodies

Key to the management of foreign bodies is the understanding that different foreign bodies require different interventions. The first separation is whether the material is a true foreign body or a food impaction. The latter being the most common type of foreign body in adult gastroenterology. It should be recognized that if a bone is present in the swallowed food bolus, it is no longer a food impaction but a true foreign body. Further classification of a foreign body is based on its characteristics: round, sharp, or unique. Round objects include coins or buttons; sharp objects include bones and safety pins; and unique objects include button batteries or body bagging of narcotics.

Food Impaction

Food impaction is one of the most common reasons for urgent endoscopy. These are typically older adults who can relate the exact time and nature of swallowed material. They may relate a history of prior episodes of either impaction or intermittent dysphagia. Food bolus impactions particularly predispose patients to complete esophageal obstruction manifested by inability to tolerate secretions. If the nature of the material is deemed not to contain any bones, the routine radiography studies are not required. Excess saliva should be removed from the esophagus prior to intubation. The material is often meat or bread. The material is manipulated with devices passed endoscopically. The key is that the material should not be blindly pushed into the stomach. The material could be endoscopically removed, or the scope can pass around the bolus and enter the stomach, followed by the bolus itself. Most patients will have some form of distal esophageal pathology (e.g., Schatzki's ring, peptic stricture, or eosinophilic esophagitis) to explain the impaction. Extreme care should be employed if the use of a meat tenderizer or gas forming agents is contemplated in the management of patient with food impaction; however, both carry the risk of perforation. Given the widespread availability of endoscopy, many authorities consider these techniques inappropriate in the current management of food impaction. Figure 10.1 shows endoscopic appearances of food impaction in the esophagus.

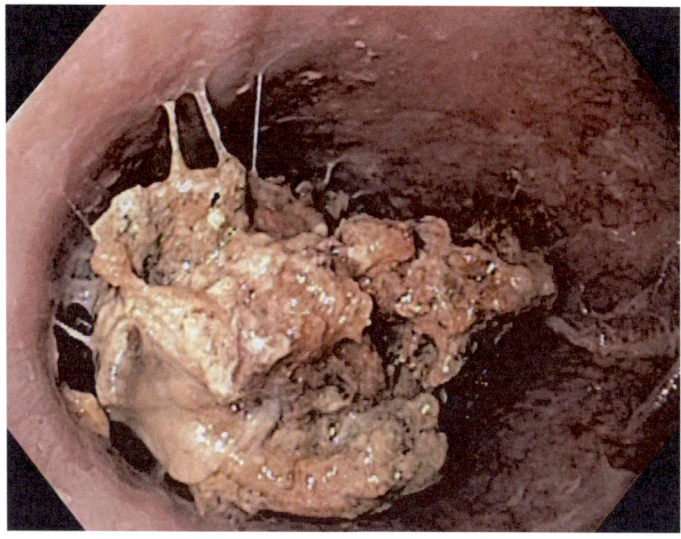

FIGURE 10.1 Endoscopic appearances of food impaction in the esophagus. Patient with known achalasia, previously treated with Heller myotomy, presents to endoscopy with symptoms of food impaction after ingesting meat the night before during a meal. Roth net was used to retrieve the impacted meat in the esophagus

Round Foreign Bodies

The majority of round foreign bodies are seen in children, although intoxicated adults may also swallow coins. Most coins, if passed into the stomach, will pass through the remainder of the gastrointestinal tract. In children, the small diameter of the esophagus may lead to proximal impaction. All coins remaining in the esophagus should be removed. A variety of methods have been reported to help remove coins from the esophagus. No matter which method is chosen, it is critical that the physician is prepared to protect patients' airways. Children with esophageal foreign bodies may present with airway obstruction.

Sharp Foreign Bodies

A host of sharp foreign bodies or objects may be ingested. Perhaps the two most common are the safety pin and dental bridge. These objects should be removed as soon as possible. In many situations, this can be done endoscopically. Airway protection and surgical backup should be available. The long-standing principle to remember when removing sharp foreign bodies is that leading edges perforate, trailing edges do not. In other words, the safety pin should be removed with the sharp edge trailing by grabbing it at the circular blunt end. In most situations, further protection can be obtained by having a hood over the entire object. See Fig. 10.2 for the endoscopic appearance of fishbone in the esophagus and stomach.

Unique Foreign Bodies

The button battery represents the best example in a category of unique foreign bodies. Unless a lateral radiograph is obtained, the AP view may look like a coin, resulting in a delay in removal. On lateral films, the button battery presents as a double density because of its bilaminar design. Button batter-

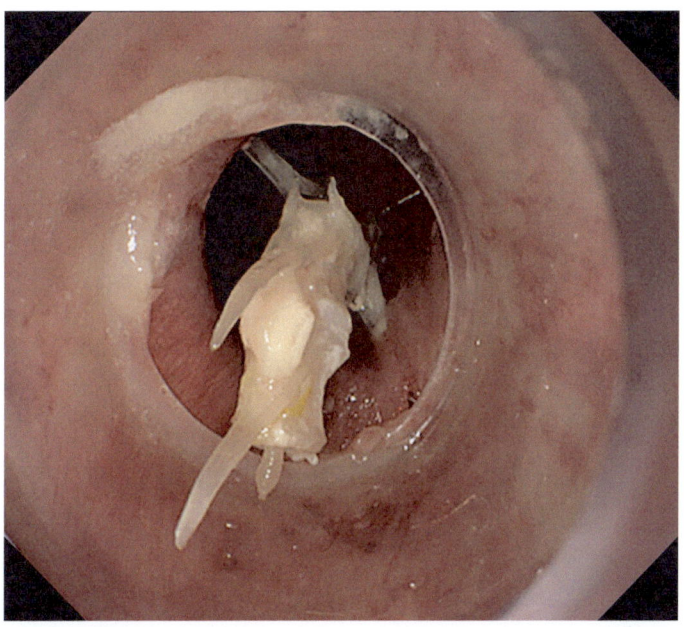

Figure 10.2 Endoscopic appearance of fishbone in the esophagus

ies should be removed as soon as possible. They produce three types of injury: (1) pressure necrosis, common to all foreign bodies, (2) electrical injury, and (3) caustic injury due to presence of alkaline materials in the battery. Injury related to the button batteries can lead to fistula formation, erosion in to the aorta, and death. A button battery in the esophagus requires urgent removal, as the alkaline substance act rapidly on the esophageal mucosa. In the long run, injury related to button batteries may lead to difficult-to-manage esophageal strictures. For a long time, there was a disagreement about the best approach to remove button batteries. Many could not be removed endoscopically. At present, the technique of choice is the use of a basket (Roth), which was originally designed to remove polyps or fragments of a polyp. It is highly recommended that every emergency endoscopy cart should be equipped with this basket. See Fig. 10.3 for endoscopic appearance of PTP (packaging for tablets) sheet in the esophagus.

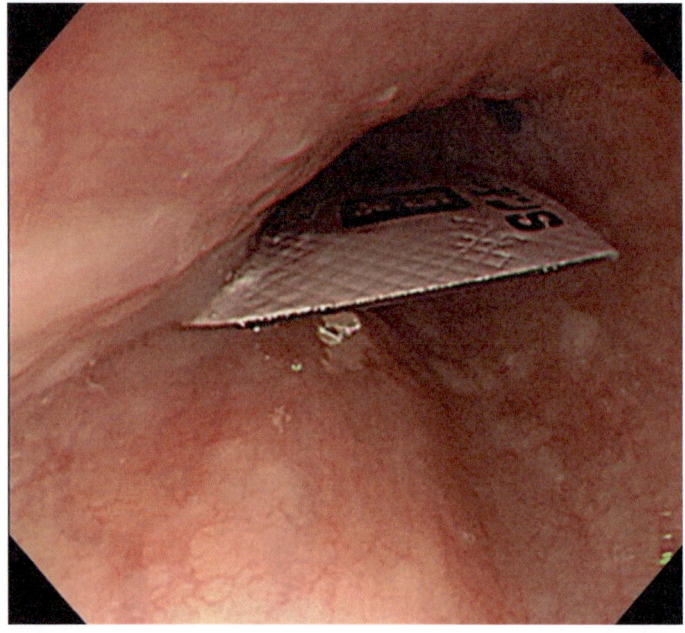

Figure 10.3 Endoscopic appearance of Press Through Packages (PTP) sheet in the esophagus

Body Packing

Body packing refers to the ingestion of narcotics in packets that ultimately pass the gastrointestinal tract. If identified anywhere in the gastrointestinal tract, there should be no attempt to remove them endoscopically. See Fig. 10.4 for radiographic imaging of a patient who ingested heroine packets [1]. If the packet is broken, it will release the contained drugs. If cocaine is present, it can result in death, since no antidote is available. Patients should be admitted and observed, with frequent urine and serum drug screens to assess for leakage of drug from the packets. Surgical intervention is indicated if intestinal obstruction or signs of suspected rupture occur.

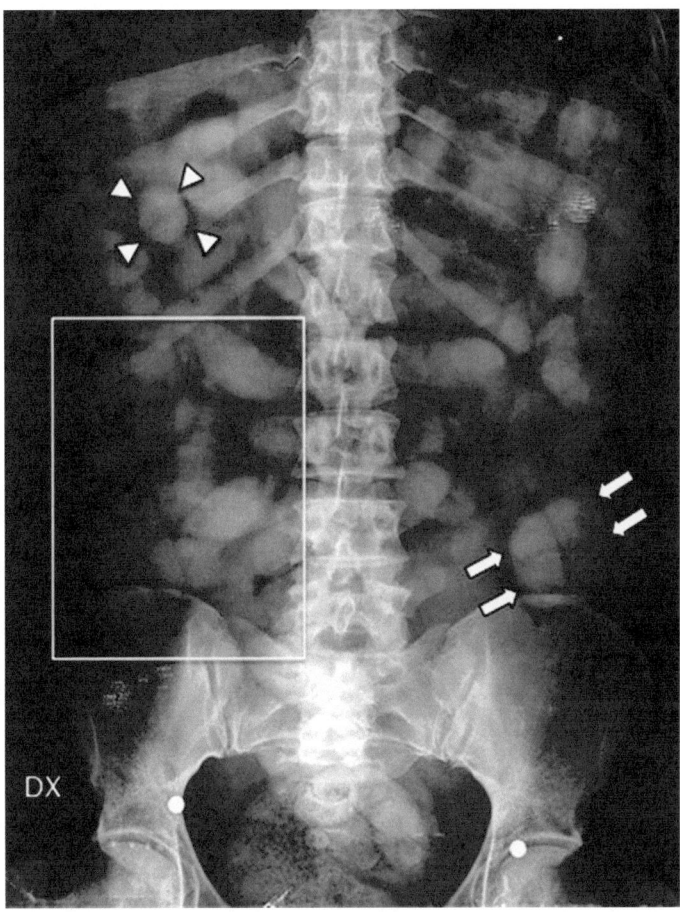

FIGURE 10.4 Radiographic study showing drug body packing. Plain abdominal film showing typical findings in body packing practice: the double-condom sign is seen as lucent rims around dense packets (arrowheads), the parallelism sign defined as firm packages aligning parallel to each other in the bowel lumen (arrows), and the tictac sign (in the white box). (With permission from Sica et al. [1])

Reference

1. Sica G, Guida F, Bocchini G, et al. Imaging of drug smuggling by body packing. Semin Ultrasound CT MR. 2015;36:39–47.

Chapter 11
Gastroesophageal Reflux Disease (GERD)

Introduction

As per the Montreal classification, GERD is classified into esophageal or extra-esophageal syndromes. Esophageal syndromes are further subdivided into whether symptoms or esophageal injury are present: (1) symptomatic syndromes, typical reflux syndrome, and reflux chest pain syndrome, and (2) syndromes with esophageal injury, reflux esophagitis, reflux stricture, Barrett's esophagus, and esophageal adenocarcinoma. Extra-esophageal syndromes are divided into established GERD-related conditions and those that are possibly associated: (1) established associations, reflux cough syndrome, reflux laryngitis syndrome, reflux asthma syndrome, and reflux dental erosions syndrome, and (2) proposed associations, pharyngitis, sinusitis, idiopathic pulmonary fibrosis, and recurrent otitis media. See Fig. 11.1 for a diagram of the Montreal classification of GERD [1].

GERD Phenotypes

GERD patients can be further classified into one of three phenotypes: (1) nonerosive reflux disease (NERD), (2) erosive esophagitis (EE), and (3) Barrett's esophagus (see Fig. 11.2 for the endoscopic appearance of these GERD

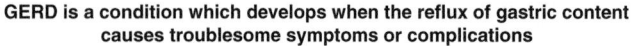

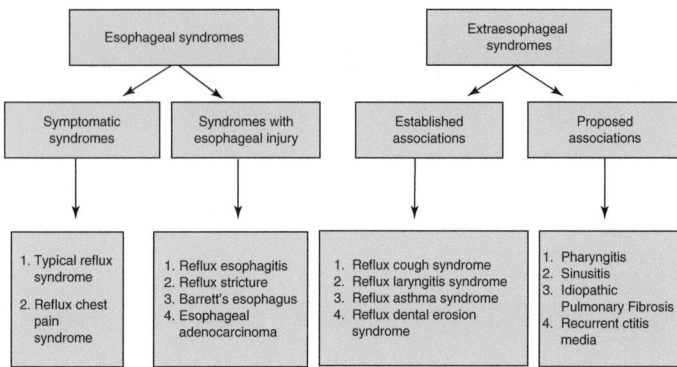

Figure 11.1 Montreal classification of GERD. The overall definition of GERD and its constituent syndromes. (With permission from Vakil et al. [1])

phenotypes). Both NERD and EE have different pathophysiological mechanisms, prognosis, and response to GERD treatment with PPI or H2 blockers. NERD accounts for the majority of GERD patients, with recent data suggesting that 70% of the GERD population have NERD. Up to 50% of heartburn patients with normal upper endoscopy show acid exposure within the physiological range. NERD patients demonstrate a 30–40% symptomatic response rate to once daily PPI therapy, while up to 60% of EE patients report improvement on therapy. The recent Rome IV classification of functional esophageal disorders defines the group of patients with normal acid exposure who are responsive to PPI therapy and demonstrate positive symptom index to reflux episodes as patients with reflux hypersensitivity. See Functional Esophageal Disorders section for further information. Esophageal hypersensitivity in addi-

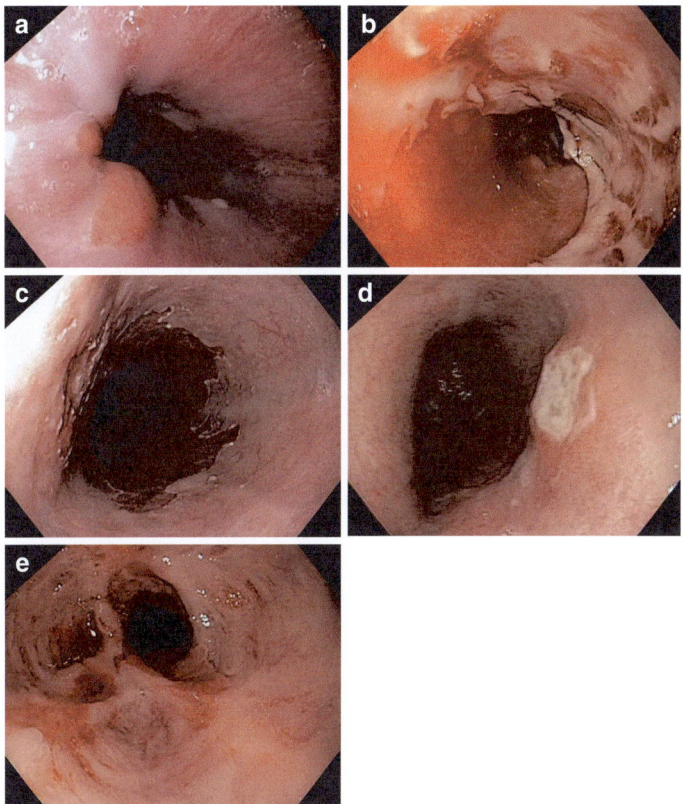

FIGURE 11.2 Endoscopic appearance of GERD manifestations and complications. (**a**) NERD, (**b**) erosive esophagitis, (**c**) Barrett's esophagus, (**d**) esophageal ulcer, (**e**) esophageal stricture. Gastroesophageal reflux disease has a spectrum of endoscopic appearances. A normal appearing esophagus (nonerosive reflux disease (NERD), **a**), inflammation of the esophagus (erosive esophagitis (EE), **b**), premalignant lesion of the esophagus (Barrett's esophagus, **c**), ulceration of the esophagus (**d**), and stricture formation from long-standing inflammation/ulceration (esophageal stricture – **e**)

tion to esophageal acid exposure is postulated to play an important role in symptom generation of NERD patients and may explain the difference in response rate between NERD and EE patients.

Pathophysiology

Gastroesophageal reflux disease (GERD) is defined as the reflux of gastric contents back into the esophagus. There are three main underlying mechanisms that can result in GERD. In healthy subjects, reflux of gastric contents primarily occurs in the postprandial period (physiologic reflux) due to transient lower esophageal sphincter relaxation (TLESR). This is a vagally mediated reflex that occurs in response to fundic distension, thus triggering a transient relaxation of the lower esophageal sphincter (LES). The hallmark of the TLESR is that the LES relaxes to gastric baseline pressure in the absence of preceding primary or secondary peristalsis. This creates a common cavity that favors the movement of material from the abdomen into the thoracic cavity, since intra-abdominal pressure exceeds intrathoracic baseline pressure. TLESR is a physiologic event that is responsible for venting swallowed air and accounts for almost all reflux events in healthy subjects and 55–80% of reflux events in patients with GERD. The other important mechanisms that may result in gastroesophageal reflux include a low baseline LES pressure and stress reflux. The latter is indicative of LES inability to mount a sufficient pressure to prevent reflux from occurring in response to a sudden increase in intra-abdominal pressure. However, other pathophysiological mechanisms also have a role in GERD, such as hiatal hernia, esophageal dysmotility, delayed gastric emptying, duodenogastroesophageal reflux, impaired defense mechanisms, decrease in salivation, and others. See Fig. 11.3 for summary of GERD pathophysiological mechanisms [2].

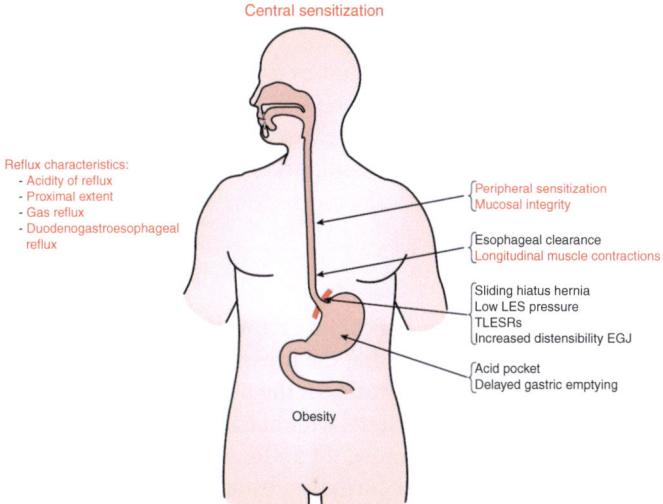

Figure 11.3 Pathophysiological mechanisms of GERD. Overview of the factors which play a role in the provocation and perception of reflux. The factors which provoke or increase reflux are illustrated in black, while the factors which influence perception are shown in red. (With permission from Herregods et al. [2])

The Anti-reflux Barrier

Dysfunction of the anti-reflux barrier is considered to be the most important factor in the pathophysiology of GERD. It is accepted that the major elements of anti-reflux barrier are the lower esophageal sphincter (LES) and the diaphragm. The LES is a thickened ring of circular smooth muscle located at the distal 2–3 cm of the esophagus and serves as the mechanical barrier that prevents reflux of acid and pepsin from the stomach back into the esophagus. The right crus of the diaphragm encircles the LES and provides additional mechanical support. Previous studies proposed that patients with GERD have higher rates of TLESR than healthy controls. However, most recent studies found no increased rate of TLESR in patients with GERD. It was demonstrated that TLESRs were more likely to be associated with acid reflux in patients with GERD when compared to healthy volunteers.

Hiatal Hernia

Hiatal hernia is another important factor in the pathogenesis of GERD. It has been shown that the prevalence and size of hiatal hernia increase with the severity of the disease. See Fig. 11.4 for hiatal hernia types [3]. Patients with hiatal hernia had a greater sensitivity to the induction of TLESRs in response to fundic distention. This has been further substantiated by data from ambulatory esophageal manometry showing GERD patients with hiatal hernias to have a substantial increase in the number of reflux episodes during swallow-induced LES relaxations [4]. In addition, hiatal hernias are associated with delayed esophageal clearance by promoting retrograde flow across the esophagogastric junction during swallow-induced LES relaxation. This effect is more pronounced in patients with a nonreducible hernia. Thus, the presence of a nonreducible hiatal hernia disrupts the sphincter mechanism and prolongs esophageal clearance, leading to increase in esophageal acid exposure time.

Esophageal Dysmotility

Patients with impaired esophageal motility have more severe gastroesophageal reflux, slower acid clearance time, worse mucosal injury, and more frequent extra-esophageal manifestations of GERD. While the majority of GERD patients have normal esophageal motility, a variety of esophageal motility abnormalities have been described in GERD patients. They include hypotensive LES, ineffective esophageal motility (IEM), absent contractility, jackhammer esophagus, distal esophageal spasm, and abnormal secondary peristalsis. A retrospective analysis of 600 conventional manometric tracings

Esophageal Dysmotility 91

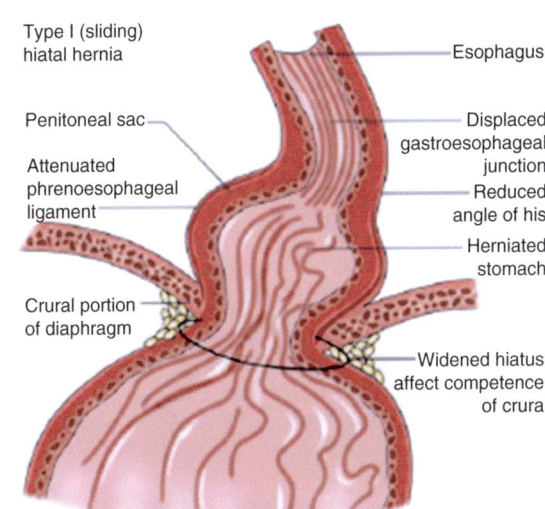

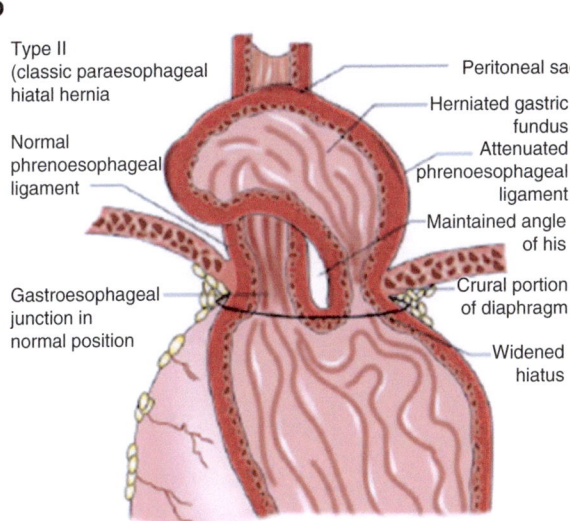

FIGURE 11.4 Hiatal hernia types. (**a**) Type 1, sliding hiatal hernia; (**b**) type II, true paraesophageal hernia; (**c**) type III, mixed paraesophageal hernia; (**d**) type IV, (giant) paraesophageal hernia. (With permission from Jeur [3])

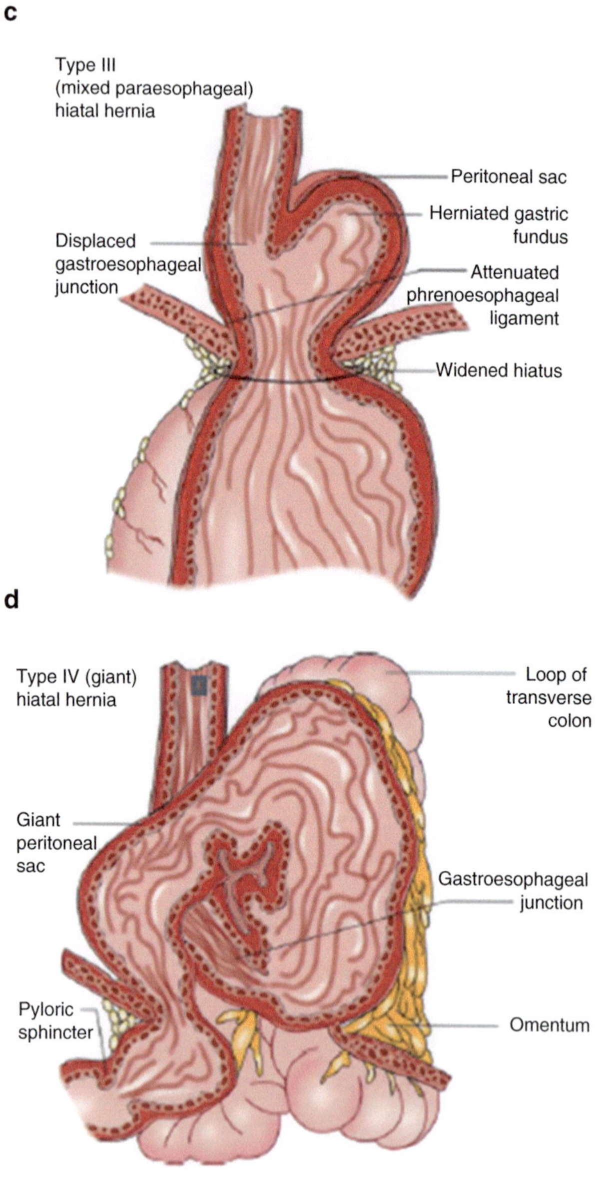

Figure 11.4 (continued)

identifies 61 patients with ineffective esophageal motility, defined by the occurrence of low amplitude (<30 mmHg) contractions during at least 30% of the swallows. Patients with IEM, as defined above, have prolonged esophageal acid clearance in both the upright and recumbent positions. The importance of esophageal dysmotility in the pathogenesis of GERD is best illustrated by scleroderma. Esophageal involvement is the most common gastrointestinal manifestation of scleroderma. In scleroderma, severe pathophysiological mechanisms contribute to the development of GERD, including hypotensive LES and impaired or absent esophageal peristalsis. Furthermore, many patients with scleroderma have an associated sicca syndrome and therefore have reduced acid neutralization capacity as a result of the absence of saliva. Abnormal esophageal motility appears to be less common in nonerosive reflux disease (NERD) and more common in patients with erosive esophagitis or Barrett's esophagus.

Gastric Acid Secretion

There is no evidence to suggest that GERD patients suffer from hypersecretion of gastric acid. However, in patients with moderate to severe corpus gastritis, eradication of *Helicobacter pylori* (*H. pylori*) may improve gastric hyposecretion and lead to significant gastroesophageal reflux in those with pre-existing, subclinical impaired gastroesophageal barrier. Patients with Zollinger-Ellison syndrome, who demonstrate gastric hypersecretion of acid, appear to have an increased risk for GERD.

Duodenogastroesophageal Reflux

Duodenogastroesophageal reflux by itself may not cause significant damage to the esophageal mucosa, but it may act synergistically with acid to produce esophagitis and may be responsible for typical GERD symptoms. It is composed primarily of pepsin, bile, acids, and trypsin. Ambulatory 24-h esophageal pH monitoring and Bilitec 2000 (a spectrophotometric system that measures bilirubin concentration within the esophagus, independent of pH) in patients with GERD showed that 28% of heartburn episodes were associated with acid reflux, 6–9% with duodenogastroesophageal reflux, and 12% with mixed acid and duodenogastroesophageal reflux. However, 51% of heartburn episodes occurred in the absence of gastroesophageal reflux. Gastric surgery, which predisposes subjects to duodenogastroesophageal reflux, is not associated with an increased risk of esophageal mucosal injury compared with controls. Furthermore, severe injury to the esophageal mucosa is more associated with combination of duodenogastroesophageal and acid reflux than duodenogastroesophageal reflux alone. Regardless, duodenogastroesophageal reflux appears to be least common in NERD patients and most common in patients with long segment Barrett's esophagus. Recent studies have also suggested that duodenogastroesophageal reflux plays an important role in symptom generation of patients with refractory GERD.

Non-acid Reflux

Approximately 50% of GERD patients who remain symptomatic with GERD symptoms on double-dose PPI demonstrate non-acidic reflux as the underlying cause, defined as pH >4 on pH-impedance testing (weakly acidic pH 4–7, weakly alkaline >7). It is proposed that both esophageal hypersensitivity and reflux-related mechanical distension of the esophagus may play a role in symptom generation with this type of reflux. Patients with negative pH test but positive impedance for weakly acidic reflux and associated symptoms are characterized as having reflux hypersensitivity, per Rome IV criteria. In addition, proximal esophageal migration of non-acid reflux as well as the presence of gas in the refluxate leads to increase likelihood of symptoms generation in refractory GERD patients. This may be due to increased sensitivity to mechanical stimulation at the esophageal transition zone between smooth and striated muscles, compared to the distal esophagus.

Dilated Intercellular Spaces

The healthy esophagus is covered with squamous epithelium, a tight barrier which prevents noxious stimuli from passing from the lumen to the mucosa where they can activate peripheral nocioreceptors. Studies using transmission electron microscopy have demonstrated that acid perfusion into the lower part of the esophagus of rabbit models result in dilated intercellular spaces (DIS) in the esophageal epithelium. It has been shown that both acid and non-acidic reflux can cause these morphological changes regardless if esophagitis is present or absent. Interestingly, reflux exposure in the distal esophagus has been also associated with proximal esophageal DIS. It has been postulated that DIS are caused by increased mucosal permeability and subsequent ionic flow through the epithelium. Water subsequently flows down this osmotic-driven gradient into the DIS resulting in dilation. In addition, increased mucosal permeability secondary to increased rates of proteolytic cleavage of cell to cell adhesion proteins (i.e., e-cadherin) further adds to weakening of the epithelial acid barrier. Mucosal permeability changes can be further evaluated by multichannel intraluminal impedance monitoring or mucosal impedance [5]. Low esophageal baseline impedance values have been shown to be associated with increased esophageal acid exposure and thus the presence of DIS's. In contrast, PPI therapy or surgical/endoscopic fundoplication have been associated with increase in baseline impedance values in GERD patients.

Many believe that DIS is a biomarker for GERD that may be reversible with PPI therapy. Interestingly, most healthy control patients with DIS did not experience symptoms of GERD. It remains to be elucidated whether the presence of DIS correlates with symptoms of GERD, as other studies have shown similar results with no correlation between the two. See Fig. 11.5 for an example of a transmission electron microscope picture of a dilated intracellular space [6].

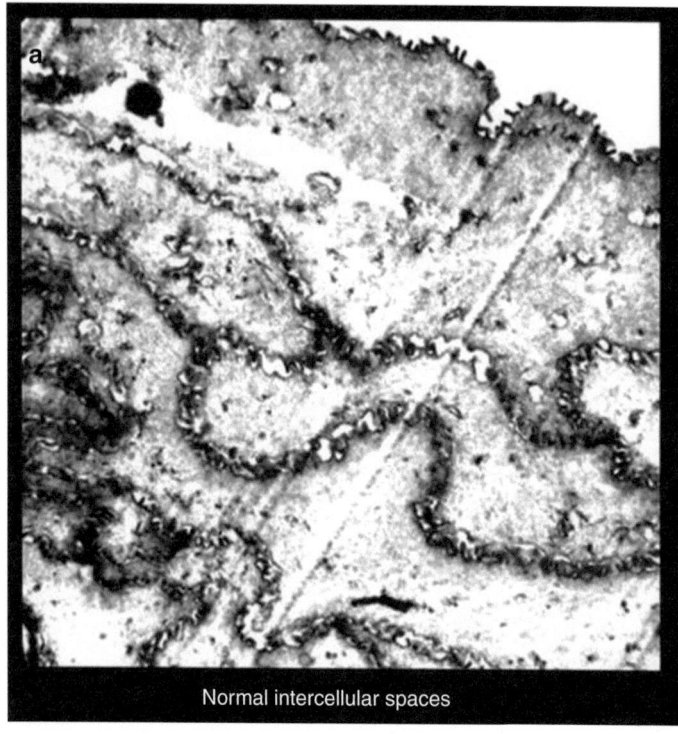

FIGURE 11.5 Dilated intercellular spaces. Transmission electron microscopy photographs of the esophageal biopsies showing normal diameter intercellular space (**a**) in a healthy patient (mean ~0.33 μm) and dilated intercellular spaces in a patient with NERD (**b**) (mean ~0.92 μm). (Original magnification X3000). (With permission from Orlando et al. [6])

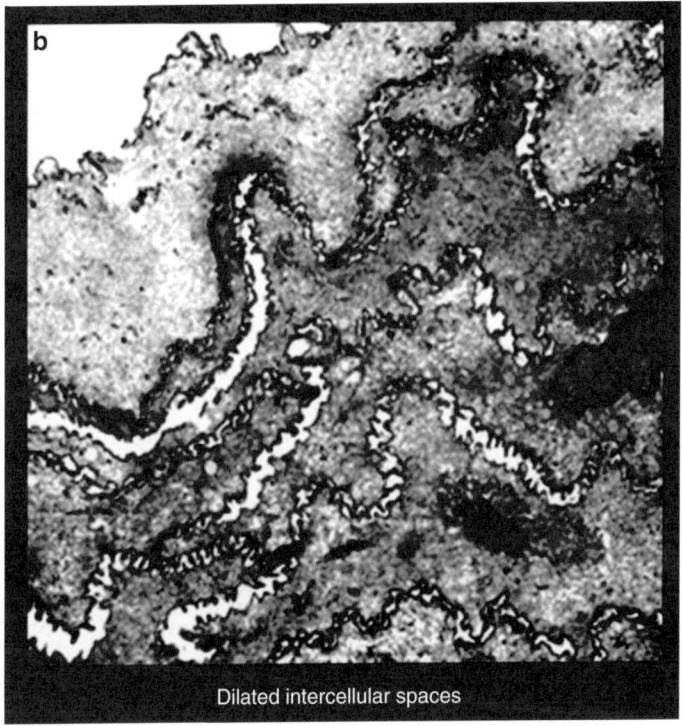

FIGURE 11.5 (continued)

However, in a recent small study, Dunbar et al. assessed 12 patients with severe reflux esophagitis who achieved complete healing on PPI therapy [7]. The authors then discontinued PPI treatment and followed the patients weekly with repeat esophageal biopsies demonstrating T-lymphocyte-predominant esophageal inflammation and basal cell and papillary hyperplasia without loss of surface cells. The results of this study suggest that the pathogenesis of erosive esophagitis is cytokine-mediated rather than chemical injury from acid reflux.

Esophageal Hypersensitivity

PPI nonresponders, NERD, functional heartburn, and those with reflux hypersensitivity have consistently demonstrated decreased perception thresholds for pain with either esophageal balloon distension, acid perfusion, or electrical stimulation, as compared with patients with erosive esophagitis or Barrett's esophagus. Both peripheral and central sensitization play important roles in esophageal hypersensitivity in these patients. Peripheral sensitization to esophageal stimuli may be related to excessive stimulation of afferent nerve receptors, which result in release of intracellular inflammatory mediators, increased expression of additional peripheral receptors, and subsequent decrease threshold for nerve transduction. This is thought to cause sensitization at the site of injury. Receptors that have been implicated in esophageal peripheral sensitization include acid sensitivity ion channels, purinergic receptors (P2X), and transient receptor vanilloid 1 (TRPV) receptors. The expression of the TRPV-1 receptor has been shown to specifically increase in inflamed esophageal mucosa tissue with activation associated with release of calcitonin gene-activating factor, substance P, and platelet-activating factor. Both substance P and platelet-activating factor are thought to be vital in promoting additional inflammation, increased mucosal permeability, and further peripheral sensitization.

Gastric Dysmotility

Approximately 20% of patients with GERD may have delayed gastric emptying, but there is no direct correlation between degree of gastric dysmotility and severity of GERD. It has been postulated that in patients with delayed gastric emptying, postprandial gastric distension may lead to increased triggering of TLESRs leading to episodes of gastroesophageal reflux. However, a recent study demonstrated that delayed gastric emptying, despite being associated with increased number of daily and postprandial reflux events, was not associated with increased esophageal acid exposure.

Genetic Factors

Genetic factors implicated in GERD include (1) family history of GERD, (2) increased concordance of symptoms in monozygotic twins compared with dizygotic twins (42% vs 26%, respectively), and (3) disease of the esophagus or stomach in first-degree relatives (not including spouses). Gene mapping studies conducted in pediatric GERD patients, with family history of GERD, found chromosome 13q14 to be associated with GERD symptoms. In addition, a recent study implicates collagen type III alpha (COL3A1) on chromosome 2 to be associated with familial dominant transmission of GERD in males with hiatal hernias. These aforementioned findings suggest that there may be a genetic influence beyond that of shared communal environmental factors.

The Role of *Helicobacter pylori* in GERD

There is conflicting evidence regarding the association of *Helicobacter pylori* (*H. pylori*) infection with GRD. Recent data suggest *H. pylori* infection may protect against the development of complications of GERD (e.g., Barrett's esophagus, esophageal adenocarcinoma), particularly in patients infected with cytotoxin-associated gene A (cagA+) positive strains of *H. pylori*. However, there has been conflicting data as to whether *H. pylori* infection is associated with less GERD symptoms, thereby calling into question whether the negative associations of GERD complications with *H. pylori* is related to the inhibition of gastroesophageal reflux.

Diagnosis of GERD

When heartburn is the predominant or sole symptom, gastroesophageal reflux is the underlying cause in at least 75% of individuals, indicating that the presence of heartburn is specific for the diagnosis of GERD. Other GERD-related symptoms include acid regurgitation, sour and bitter taste in mouth, water brash, dysphagia, odynophagia, chest pain, globus sensation, chronic cough, hoarseness, and wheezing.

Investigations

Diagnostic evaluation of GERD patients is not needed in most cases, and anti-reflux treatment is commonly delivered empirically. In first-time health-care seekers, diagnostic evaluation is indicated if alarm symptoms are present (dysphagia, odynophagia, anorexia, weight loss, and evidence of upper GI bleed). Presently, most physicians accept the concept that a marked symptomatic response to anti-reflux treatment is highly suggestive of GERD as the underlying cause of symptoms.

Upper Endoscopy

Upper endoscopy has a low sensitivity for the diagnosis of GERD as up to 60–70% of the patients with GERD-related symptoms have no evidence of esophageal mucosal injury on endoscopy and are defined as nonerosive reflux disease (NERD). However, upper endoscopy remains the gold standard for the diagnosis of erosive esophagitis, Barrett's esophagus, and other complications of GERD, such as ulceration and stricture. See Table 11.1 for classification of erosive esophagitis [8]. The test is indicated in patients with alarm symptoms and to exclude Barrett's esophagus in those with long-term GERD symptoms.

TABLE 11.1 Classification systems for erosive esophagitis. Los Angeles and Savary-Miller classification are two classification systems that are commonly used to grade severity of erosive esophagitis on upper endoscopy

Classification	Grade	Description
Los Angeles	A	One (or more) mucosal break no longer than 5 mm that does not extend between the tops of 2 mucosal folds
	B	One (or more) mucosal break >5 mm that does not extend between the tops of 2 mucosal folds
	C	One (or more) mucosal break that is continuous between the tops of ≥2 mucosal folds but that involves <75% of the circumference
	D	One (or more) mucosal break that involves at least 75% of the esophageal circumference
Savary-Miller	1	Single erosion above the gastroesophageal mucosal junction
	2	Multiple, noncircumferential erosions above the gastroesophageal mucosal junction
	3	Circumferential erosion above the mucosal junction
	4	Chronic change with esophageal ulceration and associated stricture
	5	Barrett's esophagus with histologically confirmed intestinal differentiation within the columnar epithelium

With permission from Muthusamy et al. [8]

Ambulatory 24-h Esophageal pH Monitoring

The test is positive in up to 75% of those with erosive esophagitis and 45% with nonerosive reflux disease. The test is invasive, expensive, and may not be readily available to community-based physicians. Testing should be performed off PPI therapy to document the presence or absence of abnormal esophageal acid exposure. Presently, 24-h esophageal pH monitoring is best reserved for patients with the following characteristics: (1) symptomatic patients with heartburn and with normal endoscopy; (2) patients with no history of documented GERD, who failed treatment with a PPI (off treatment); and (3) patients with atypical/extraesophageal symptoms, who are poorly responsive to adequate trial of anti-reflux therapy (off treatment).

Ambulatory esophageal pH testing can be performed with a catheter or by using the wireless technology (Bravo capsule), the latter being more commonly used these days. An abnormal pH test is whenever the percent total time pH <4 is greater than 4.2% (DeMeester score >14.72). The wireless pH capsule (Bravo) is attached 6 cm from LES after being deployed from the tip of a catheter either with or without direct visualization at the time of upper endoscopy. The wireless technology allows less patient discomfort, ability to continue with daily activity, and for long duration of pH monitoring (up to 96 h). Consequently, Bravo testing has sensitivity and clinical yield that are comparable if not better than the catheter-based pH testing. Patients are advised to be off anti-reflux medications for at least 7 days and fast for at least 6–8 h before the test. Patients are asked to keep a diary as well as press a button on the recorder device when they are having GERD symptoms. Once the placement has been completed, patients are advised to pursue their normal daily activity. Contraindications to the wireless pH capsule include strictures in the gastrointestinal tract, defibrillator or pacemaker, and scheduling of an MRI 30 days after the wireless pH capsule has been placed. pH profiles in the supine and upright positions are evaluated by the wireless pH capsule and may have clinical relevance in terms of management of patient's reflux symptoms, especially if one or the other position is predominant in causing more symptomatic reflux events. If the test is done for at least 48 h, the 24-h period the patient was most symptomatic with abnormal pH test results is used for results interpretation. A Bravo test is considered positive if the combined percent total time pH <4 is greater than 5.2%.

Assessment of symptom correlation is done with symptom index (SI) and symptom association probability (SAP) scores. SI is the percentage of reflux-related symptoms as it is related to the total number of symptoms during a 24-h period. (A positive SI is >50%). The reliability of the SI score decreases if too few or too many reflux events occur. SAP, on the other hand, compliments SI by using a two by two contingency table and the Fisher's exact test. SAP is a calculation of the probability that reflux and symptoms do not occur by chance alone. SAP is positive if it is greater than 95%. Therefore, SI and SAP complement each other, where SI calculates the strength of reflux and symptom association, while SAP aids to determine if symptom and reflux events are occurring due to chance.

Multichannel Intraluminal pH Impedance

The combination of impedance catheter and pH sensor provides a unique opportunity to assess the composition (air, liquid, mixed), direction (anterograde/retrograde), extent (proximal, distal), velocity, clearance time, and pH (acidic, weakly acidic, or weakly alkaline) of a reflux event. Ring electrodes line the 2 mm wide esophageal impedance pH catheter and are positioned at 3, 5, 7, 9, 15, and 17 cm from the EGJ junction. The pH sensor is located 5 cm above the EGJ. The esophageal impedance catheter functions based on Ohm's law; impedance to flow is inversely related to the medium's electrical conductivity characteristics. This allows for detection of various composites of contact in the esophageal lumen depending on the impedance characteristics. For example, a liquid reflux episode will show a greater than 50% drop in mucosal impedance and then a rise to baseline as it moves proximally up the esophagus. Gas is considered to have a low electrical conductivity and therefore is indicated as an increase in luminal impedance.

The multichannel intraluminal impedance is an important tool for the assessment of symptomatic patients with heartburn or acid regurgitation who failed PPI twice daily, patients with atypical GERD symptoms, evaluation of GERD in patients before lung transplantation, and evaluation of patients with excessive belching and rumination syndrome. Studies have demonstrated the role of weakly acidic reflux in generating GERD symptoms in these challenging patient populations. Overall, residual acid reflux is a very uncommon cause of symptoms in patients who failed PPI twice daily. The pH-impedance testing is useful in stratifying PPI failure patients as those having reflux hypersensitivity or functional heartburn (Fig. 11.6) [9]. Other uses for

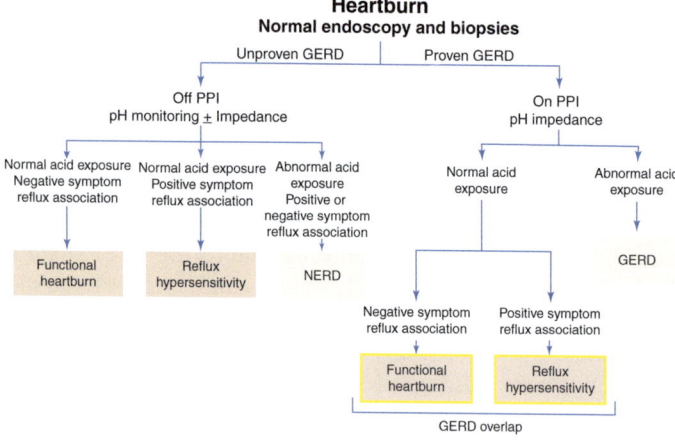

FIGURE 11.6 Defining GERD, functional heartburn, and reflux hypersensitivity based on pH-impedance testing. Further classification of patients with heartburn and no evidence of esophagitis at endoscopy using pH monitoring or pH impedance. The figure shows classification categories by findings and is not meant to suggest a diagnostic management algorithm for use in clinical practice. (With permission from Aziz et al. [9])

pH-impedance testing include (1) impedance assessment of bolus transit within the esophageal lumen allowing for improved characterization of patients with esophageal motility disorders with predominant complaint of dysphagia, (2) detection of liquid and gas composites, in patients with excessive belching or rumination syndrome, and (3) evaluation of mucosal integrity in patients with chronic GERD (impedance baseline levels).

The test provides traditional pH parameters, including percent time pH <4 in the supine and upright position as well as total time regardless of position. The pH parameter remains the most reliable in predicting patient's outcome with a given intervention such as surgery or medical therapy. Impedance of acidic, weakly acidic, or weakly alkaline reflux is provided as well as liquid, gas, or mixed (gas and liquid). Reflux events are recorded in the supine and upright positions and are totaled for each type of reflux event. Manual review of the impedance test should be done, as the computer program oftentimes overestimates reflux episodes. Total reflux events are used to determine positive or negative impedance test, rather than specific positions off or on PPI.

Mucosal Impedance

Mucosal impedance (MI) is a newer technology that employs a catheter containing two sensors, which is introduced through a working channel of the endoscope at the time of endoscopy. The tip of the catheter, which contains the sensors, comes in contact with the esophageal mucosa at various increments along the esophagus to obtain real-time mucosal impedance measurements. Early results from the use of MI indicate that the technology is useful in separating between GERD and functional heartburn patients. Presently, the technique is primarily used for research purposes.

Extra-Esophageal Syndromes of GERD

There has been an increased awareness of the possible associations of GERD and a variety of extra-esophageal syndromes. Diagnosis of extra-esophageal manifestations of GERD requires a high clinical suspicion. Symptoms during sleep or after meals, the presence of typical GERD symptoms (heartburn and acid regurgitation), and adult onset of symptoms should alert the physician that GERD may be the underlying cause. The extra-esophageal manifestations of GERD originate from the oropharynx, larynx, and pulmonary system. As per the Montreal classification of GERD, established associations include reflux cough syndrome, reflux laryngitis syndrome, reflux asthma syndrome, and reflux dental erosion syndrome. Proposed associations with GERD include pharyngitis, sinusitis, globus, idiopathic pulmonary fibrosis, otitis media, sleep apnea, sleep disturbances, and cardiac arrhythmia. Unfortunately, there is no sensitive or specific test that can identify if these types of symptoms are related to GERD. If the symptoms are associated with alarm symptoms, then malignancy should be excluded. Referral to ENT is certainly indicated in patients with laryngeal, pharyngeal, or oral symptoms and to a pulmonologist in those with pulmonary-related symptoms. Laryngeal pathologies with symptoms overlapping that of GERD are listed in Table 11.2 [10].

Diagnosis of laryngeal reflux cannot be reliably made solely by findings on laryngoscopy. Findings that are highly suggestive of LPR include vocal cord polyps, pharyngeal ulceration, Eustachian tube dysfunction, and dental enamel loss to name a few. The exact frequency of these events is unknown. Only about 25% of patients with LPR will have evidence of esophageal mucosa injury at the time of endoscopy.

GERD is considered to be the third most common cause of chronic cough in adults. Patients with chronic cough pre-

TABLE 11.2 Alternative laryngopharyngeal pathologies with symptoms overlapping with those attributed to extra-esophageal reflux and their laryngoscopic findings

Pathology	EER-associated symptoms	Typical laryngoscopy findings
Muscle tension dysphonia	Hoarseness, globus, throat pain, dysphagia	No vocal fold lesions
		Superglottic hyperfunction
Vocal fold paralysis/paresis	Hoarseness, cough, dysphagia, dyspnea	Immobile or hypomobile vocal fold
	Globus	Glottic insufficiency
		Ipsilateral vocal fold atrophy ± bowing
		Supraglottic hyperfunction[a]
Presbylaryngis	Hoarseness, cough, globus	Bilateral vocal fold bowing
		Glottic insufficiency
		Supraglottic hyperfunction[a]
Irritable larynx syndrome	Cough, globus, hoarseness	Normal laryngoscopy (typical)
		Vocal fold erythema/edema
Cancer	Throat pain, hoarseness, cough, dysphagia	Mass in pharynx or larynx ± superficial ulceration
	Dyspnea, globus, ear pain	Vocal fold leukoplakia

(continued)

TABLE 11.2 (continued)

Pathology	EER-associated symptoms	Typical laryngoscopy findings
		Vocal fold hypomobility (if joint involved)
Recurrent respiratory papillomatosis	Hoarseness, cough, dyspnea, globus	Sessile or pedunculated fungiform mass in larynx/trachea
		Red stippling or vascular stalks within lesion
Laryngotracheal stenosis	Hoarseness, dyspnea	Narrowing at supraglottis, glottis, subglottis, or trachea
		Scarring at site of stenosis ± erythema
Phonotraumatic lesion	Hoarseness	Nodule, polyp, cyst, fibrous mass on vibratory edge
		Glottic insufficiency
		Supraglottic hyperfunction[a]
Vocal fold hemorrhage	Hoarseness	Submucosal hemorrhage
		Ipsilateral vocal fold edema/erythema
Polypoid corditis	Hoarseness, cough, globus, ± dyspnea	Polypoid changes of entire vocal fold epithelium

TABLE 11.2 (continued)

Pathology	EER-associated symptoms	Typical laryngoscopy findings
		Hyperdynamic mucosa
Vocal fold scarring	Hoarseness	Vocal fold sulcus
		Supraglottic hyperfunction
Vocal process granuloma	Throat pain (often ipsilateral), hoarseness	Lesion or ulceration at arytenoid vocal process
	Cough, globus	Glottic insufficiency (depending on size)
		Supraglottic hyperfunction[a]
Laryngeal candidiasis	Throat pain, hoarseness, cough, dysphagia	White speckling of fungus in pharynx and larynx
	Globus	Laryngeal erythema ± ulcerations
Zenker's diverticulum	Regurgitation, hoarseness, dysphagia	Normal laryngoscopy (typical)
	Globus	Food debris in left pyriform sinus
Paradoxic vocal fold motion	Dyspnea	Normal laryngoscopy at rest
		Laryngospasm with triggers (e.g., scents, exercise)

With permission from Francis and Vaezi [10]
[a]Compensatory muscle tension dysphonia

sumed to be due to acid reflux should be treated with high dose PPI (double dose) therapy for at least 2 months. Randomized controlled trials have shown no difference in symptom resolution when once daily or twice daily PPI were compared with placebo. A similar therapeutic approach is used in patients with hoarseness, where up to 40% of the patients have evidence of esophageal inflammation despite not having typical symptoms of GERD. In large randomized placebo controlled trial, there was no difference between twice daily PPI therapy (esomeprazole 40 mg) versus placebo in controlling hoarseness.

Up to 77% of asthmatics report GERD-related symptoms with a large study demonstrating erosive esophagitis and esophageal stricture to be associated with pulmonary conditions such as bronchiectasis, pulmonary fibrosis, and chronic obstructive pulmonary disease. Up to 35% of asthmatics have been shown to have an abnormal esophageal acid exposure on 24-h pH study. Two main mechanisms are responsible for pulmonary involvement in GERD patients: micro aspirations of acid, which may result in bronchospasm and a vasovagal reflex. The value of PPI therapy in improving asthma symptoms has been mixed, with some studies indicating improvement in pulmonary function and decrease in use of on-demand therapy for active asthma symptoms, while others have shown no difference in asthma symptoms when PPIs have been compared to placebo.

Assessment for GERD in patients with extra-esophageal manifestations is commonly triggered by ENT examination revealing laryngopharyngeal reflux (LPR) during laryngoscopy and suspicion of a pulmonologist. Upper endoscopy is commonly performed to assess for esophageal mucosal injury. If unrevealing, in patients of PPI treatment, the catheter-based pH test or the wireless pH capsule is performed. In patients, who failed at least twice daily PPI, an impedance+pH is commonly performed on treatment.

Noncardiac Chest Pain (NCCP)

Up to 36% of patients with angina type chest pain have normal appearing coronary arteries on cardiac evaluation, thereby defining these symptoms as "noncardiac in origin." Gastroesophageal reflux disease is the most common underlying mechanism for NCCP, with prevalence ranging between 30% and 60%. The PPI test is both sensitive and specific tool in the diagnosis of GERD related NCCP. The omeprazole test is one of the most studied in GERD-related NCCP with up to 52–95% of patients reporting symptom improvement during the test as compared to 10–50% of patients receiving placebo. Patients with GERD-related NCCP are commonly treated empirically with a PPI twice daily for a period of 2 months with good response. Endoscopic therapy, using the Endocinch, has shown in one study to improve GERD-related chest pain. Patients with positive pH studies for GERD or positive PPI response treated with complete or partial fundoplication demonstrate the greatest improvement in chest pain symptoms when compared to patients without positive pH testing or PPI response prior to surgery. Esophageal motility disorders account for up to 30% of non-GERD-related NCCP, with nutcracker esophagus and hypotensive lower esophageal sphincter as the two most common findings on esophageal manometry. Smooth muscle relaxants including nifedipine, diltiazem, nitrates, and sildenafil have shown varying degrees of improvement in symptoms with therapy for spastic esophageal motility disorders (i.e., nutcracker esophagus, diffuse esophageal spasm). Many of these medications are limited from long-term use due to their various side effects. Botulinum toxin has been used in the past for treatment of NCCP in patients with spastic esophageal disorders, with up to 89% decrease in chest pain symptoms scores at 6 months; however, most often patients require repeat endoscopic injection of botulinum toxin limiting its long-term use. Peroral endoscopic myotomy (POEM) has also been used in treatment of esophageal dysmotility-related NCCP (hypercontractile disorders) with impressive initial treatment success in a few recent early trials. Esophageal hypersensitivity has been demonstrated as a major underlying mechanism for NCCP symptom generation in patients with both functional chest pain and esophageal motor disorders.

Treatment of chest pain symptoms in those with functional chest pain and those with esophageal dysmotility focuses on neuromodulators therapies using visceral analgesics. Of the tricyclic antidepressants, imipramine is the only medication that has been evaluated in a double-blind placebo controlled trial with results indicating a 52% reduction in chest pain symptoms. However, due to imipramine's side effect profile of dizziness and dry mouth, long-term use is limited. In another study, patients with incomplete chest pain symptom resolution on once daily rabeprazole and negative pH testing after 1 month of PPI treatment were treated with amitriptyline and rabeprazole once daily, with 71% of patients reporting greater than 50% global symptom improvement compared to the 26% of patients treated with double-dose rabeprazole. Venlafaxine, a serotonin norepinephrine reuptake inhibitor, also has shown promising results in treatment of noncardiac chest pain with 52% of patients describing more than 50% improvement in symptoms compared to 4% treated with placebo. In addition, sertraline, a selective serotonin receptor agonist, has shown improvement in chest pain symptoms in a small trial. On the other hand, trazodone at a dose of 50–100 mg at bedtime showed little efficacy in improving chest pain intensity and frequency compared to placebo, despite improvement in global improvement scores at 6 weeks of therapy.

Treatment with neuromodulators should follow the rule of "low and slow." Tricyclics antidepressants, for example, should be given at bedtime at a minimum dose and increased weekly to a maximum (non-mood altering) dose of 50–75 mg. Anticholinergic side effects may occur, especially in the elderly.

Alternative therapies including energy healing Johrei therapy, cognitive behavior therapy, hypnotherapy, and cop-

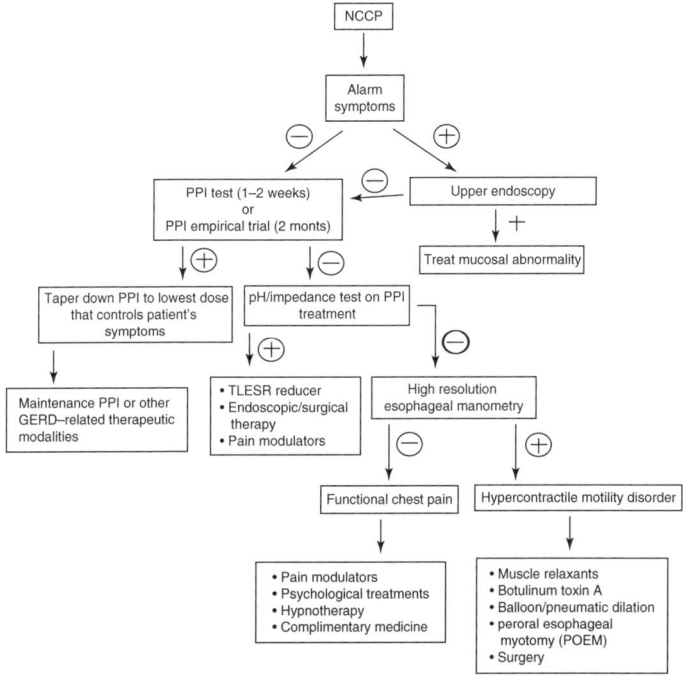

FIGURE 11.7 Management algorithm for noncardiac chest pain (NCCP). *NCCP* noncardiac chest pain, *PPI* proton pump inhibitor, *GERD* gastroesophageal reflux disease, *TLESR* transient lower esophageal sphincter relaxant. (With permission from George et al. [11])

ing skills have all shown significant improvement in chest pain intensity scores. These types of therapies may be helpful as solo or adjunctive therapies in the treatment of NCCP. See Fig. 11.7 for a management algorithm for NCCP [11].

Management of GERD

For patients with mild and infrequent reflux symptoms, it seems reasonable to use antacids and lifestyle modifications such as weight loss, cessation of smoking, sleep precautions, and elevation of the head of the bed. For patients with more severe reflux symptoms, a definitive treatment is required.

The aim of the initial GERD management includes (1) confirmation of the diagnosis of GERD, (2) adequate relief of GERD symptoms, and (3) healing of esophagitis, if present. In patients with nonerosive reflux disease (NERD), studies have demonstrated that PPIs are superior to H2 receptor antagonist (H2RA) in providing symptom relief. In patients with mild to moderate erosive esophagitis (Los Angeles Grade A and B), PPIs are superior to H2Ras in providing healing of the esophageal mucosal erosions and relieving GERD symptoms. In patients with severe erosive esophagitis (Los Angeles Grade C and D), PPIs are the sole treatment, and in some patients, even double dosing of PPI is frequently required. Failure of an 8-week course of initial therapy with a PPI should prompt a review of the diagnosis if it is solely a symptom-based diagnosis. In addition, optimization of the PPI treatment is needed and includes lifestyle modifications, improving compliance and adherence, and splitting the PPI dose. In patients who do not respond adequately to once daily PPI despite optimization of treatment, adding a second daily dose before the evening meal is a reasonable next step.

The aims of long-term management of GERD include (1) satisfactory control of symptoms, (2) maintenance of healing of erosive esophagitis, (3) prevention of relapse and complications, and (4) improvement of quality of life. As GERD is predominantly a chronic relapsing disorder, the balance of priorities for long-term care differs from that of initial therapy. PPI has been shown to be the most effective maintenance treatment of erosive esophagitis and NERD. The management options in terms of the use of PPI are either continuous daily maintenance therapy, intermittent therapy (physician's driven, predetermined course of therapy), or on-demand therapy (patient's driven, whenever symptoms occur or are expected). It has been shown that the most effective therapy was likely to be the most cost-effective one.

It is inappropriate to withdraw therapy in patients with severe erosive esophagitis (Los Angeles Grades C and D), as all patients will relapse upon cessation of therapy. For patients with mild to moderate erosive disease (Los Angeles A/B), or patients with nonerosive reflux disease, there is increasing support for an on-demand approach. The clinical value of on-demand approach has been evaluated by many studies, demonstrating proper reduction in symptoms, improved quality of life, and reduced cost.

In patients with extra-esophageal manifestations of GERD, a double-dose PPI should be offered as the initial course of therapy for a duration of up to 4 months. In patients with GERD-related NCCP, 2 months' initial treatment is recommended. In patients who demonstrate a satisfactory symptoms response, lowering the dose of PPI may be considered. Maintenance therapy is essential, and commonly the dose of PPI that induces symptom remission is likely to be the dose of PPI for long-term maintenance.

Adverse Events of Chronic PPI Treatment

There is a growing body of literature reporting the potential adverse effects of chronic PPI treatment. They include osteoporosis-associated wrist, spine, and hip fracture, nosocomial Clostridium difficile colitis, community-acquired pneumonia, small intestine bacterial overgrowth, microscopic colitis, enteric infections, traveler's diarrhea, vitamin and mineral deficiencies, ischemic heart events, dementia, renal failure, death, rebound acid secretion after PPI cessation, and fundic gland polyps. In addition, omeprazole and esomeprazole have been shown to interfere with activation of clopidogrel by CYP2C19, resulting in increased risk of an ischemic heart event, especially in patients postmyocardial infarction or stent placement. While the risk for most of the aforementioned complications is generally modest, they are more likely to occur in patients older than 50, those who take the PPI long term (>1 year) and more than once daily.

Anti-Reflux Surgery and Endoscopic Therapies

Indications for anti-reflux surgery include (1) patients with inadequate symptom control on medical therapy (with documented residual gastroesophageal reflux), (2) patients' unwillingness to take anti-reflux medications long term, (3) esophageal complications related to GERD (i.e., stricture), (4) patients with large hiatal hernia (>5 cm) and regurgitation, and (5) intolerance to side effects of medical anti-reflux treatment. Endoscopic treatment is indicated primarily in patients with inadequate symptom control on medical therapy, but with documented residual acidic reflux, and those who are not interested in medical therapy, developed side effects or allergic reaction to PPI treatment.

Surgery and endoscopic therapy are reasonable alternatives, provided the patients are fully informed about the risk and possible complications of the procedure (surgical side effects: increased flatulence, dysphagia, diarrhea, and early satiety). A long-term follow-up of patients who were randomized to medical vs surgical therapy found similar efficacy between the two therapeutic modalities. Surgical techniques include both surgical fundoplication (both complete and partial) and the LINX, a magnetic sphincter augmentation device (a ring composed from magnetic titanium beads that is placed around the lower part of the esophagus with the aim of generating an anti-reflux barrier). Studies have demonstrated that more than half of the patients who underwent surgical fundoplication were back on anti-reflux medications more than a decade later. Short-term studies have shown that the LINX procedure is highly efficacious; however, concerns remain regarding potential erosion or migration of the ring. In patients with Barrett's esophagus, surgery has not been shown to prevent the progression to dysplasia or adenocarcinoma of the esophagus.

Presently, there are two endoscopic techniques that are available to treat GERD. They include the Stretta procedure and transoral incisionless fundoplication (TIF). The Stretta technique is associated with delivery of radio-frequency energy into the lower esophagus and gastric cardia. The TIF procedure, commonly performed by surgeons, provides an anterior fundoplication (270 degree) through the scope. Both endoscopic procedures appear to be efficacious in GERD patients with small hiatal hernias (<3 cm) and without severe erosive esophagitis (Los Angeles Grades A and B).

The Refractory GERD Patient

A subset of up to 40% of the patients with heartburn demonstrates a partial or lack of response to PPI once daily. It is essential to ascertain that other pathologies mimicking GERD (heart disease in particular) are not being missed. Furthermore, poor compliance (taking the medication intermittently or on-demand) or adherence to proper time administration should be initially ruled out. PPI failure has become the most common GERD-related clinical problem that gastroenterologists and primary care physicians encounter in their practices. The current standard of care is to double the PPI dose on the assumption that most of the patients continue to have poorly controlled acid reflux for 12 weeks to assess response. However, studies have demonstrated that only an additional 25% of patients respond to such a therapeutic strategy, while the majority remain refractory to treatment. Evaluation by endoscopy and pH testing in symptomatic heartburn patients on double-dose PPI therapy is almost universally unremarkable. The next therapeutic step in these patients is dependent on the results of intraluminal pH-impedance testing [12]. This technique can identify weakly acidic and weakly alkaline reflux that may be responsible for patients' residual symptoms. About 8–10% of the refractory heartburn patients experience symptoms due to abnormal reflux and thus may benefit from a transient lower esophageal sphincter relaxation (TLESR) reducer, endoscopic therapy, or anti-reflux surgery. Patients failing double-dose PPI with normal esophageal acid exposure but positive symptom correlation (positive SI and/or SAP) with acid or non-acidic reflux events on pH-impedance testing have reflux hypersensitivity. In contrast, patients with negative symptom correlation (SI and SAP) with reflux events have functional heartburn (Fig. 11.8) [13]. Patients with reflux hypersensitivity can be treated with PPIs or neuromodulators, such as SSRIs, SNRIs, and TCAs as adjunct to PPI or solo therapy. In contrast, patients with functional heartburn benefit from treatment with neuromodulators, psychological, and alternative medicine interventions. Overall, because most heartburn patients who failed PPI twice daily have either functional heartburn or reflux hypersensitivity (>90%), it is suggestive that esophageal hypersensitivity is the main underlying mechanism of PPI failure.

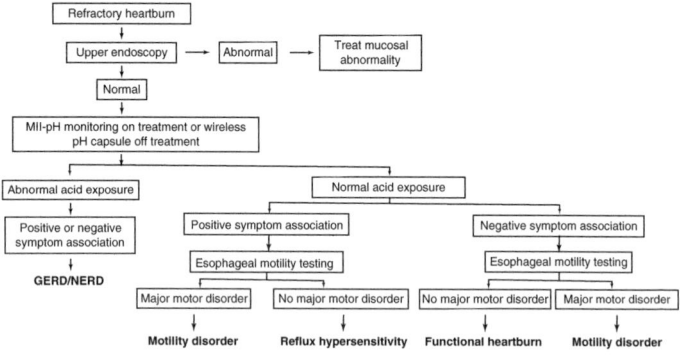

FIGURE 11.8 Diagnostic algorithm of reflux hypersensitivity and functional heartburn in refractory heartburn patients (failed PPI twice daily). GERD, gastroesophageal reflux disease; NERD, nonerosive reflux disease. (With permission from Yamasaki et al. [13])

Adjunctive therapies for refractory GERD include prokinetic agents which act to increase LES pressure, improve esophageal clearance of reflux, and increase the rate of gastric emptying. Cisapride, a medication no longer available in the US market, used in combination with H2 blockers and PPI therapy, was shown to increase the rate of esophagitis healing compared to anti-reflux therapy alone. However, the medication was found to have major side effects, especially cardiac arrhythmias due to QT prolongation which limited its use. Data regarding 5-HT4 agonists, such as mosapride and revexepride, have had mixed results regarding their efficacy as compared with placebo or PPI alone. On the other hand, two other 5-HT4 agonists, prucalopride and tegaserod, have shown some promise with early data demonstrating a decrease in the rate of reflux events, TLESRs, and esophageal acid exposure.

Centrally acting GABA receptor B agonist, baclofen, has been shown to inhibit both acidic and non-acidic reflux events, improve postprandial LES baseline pressure, and decrease the number of TLESRs compared to placebo medication. This medication can be used as an add-on therapy to PPI or as monotherapy for GERD. Most studies evaluating the efficacy of baclofen as an add-on or on-demand therapy did not show increased rate of adverse events as expected given its known neurological side effects (e.g., tiredness, dizziness, sleepiness, and accommodation disorders).

Patients with GERD not responsive to PPI therapy may be candidates for anti-reflux surgery. However, studies have indicated that partial (at least 50% improvement of symptoms) or complete response to PPI therapy in the past is the best predictor of symptom response postoperatively. Therefore, candidates for anti-reflux surgery should be carefully selected and evaluated for past response to medical treatment and for an objective evidence of GERD (esophageal inflammation on endoscopy or abnormal esophageal acid exposure on pH testing). A proposed management algorithm for patients who do not respond to PPI therapy is provided in Fig. 11.9 [14].

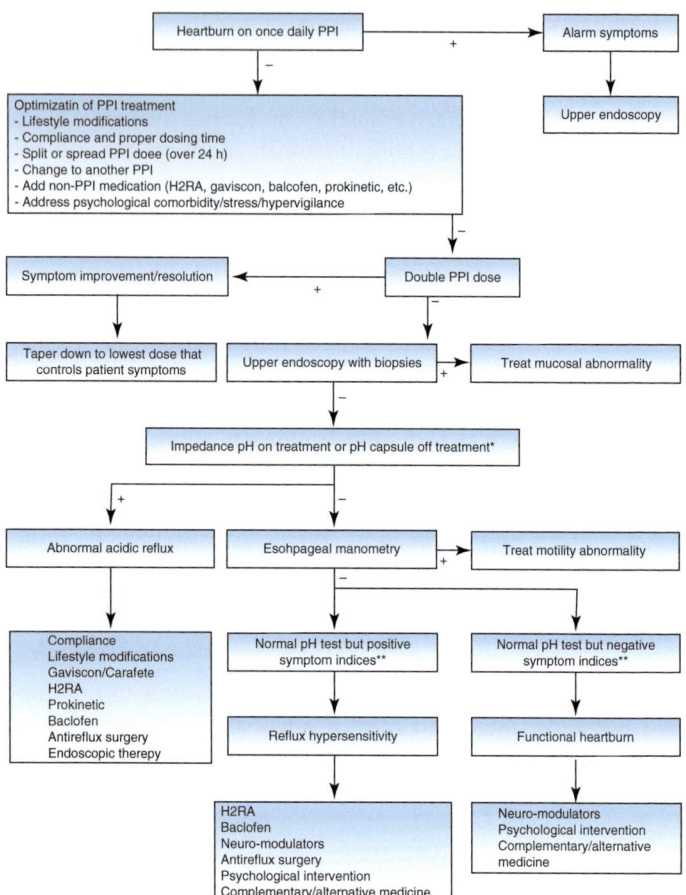

Figure 11.9 Algorithm for evaluation and management of patients who do not respond to PPI therapy. *In patients with proven GERD (abnormal pH test or erosive esophagitis), pH-impedance testing is performed on treatment; in all others (unproven GERD), pH or pH-impedance testing off treatment (prolonged wireless pH monitoring may have advantages). **With either acidic or nonacidic reflux. (With permission from Gyawali et al. [14])

References

1. Vakil N, van Zanten SV, Kahrilas P, et al. The Montreal definition and classification of gastroesophageal reflux disease: a global evidence-based consensus. Am J Gastroenterol. 2006;101:1900–20.
2. Herregods TV, Bredenoord AJ, Smout AJ. Pathophysiology of gastroesophageal reflux disease: new understanding in a new era. Neurogastroenterol Motil. 2015;27:1202–13.
3. Jeur AS. Review of literatures on laparoscopic prosthetic repair of Giant hiatal hernia than pure anatomical repair of the Crura. World J Laparosc Surg. 2010;3:85–90.
4. Kohn GP, Price RR, DeMeester SR, et al. Guidelines for the management of hiatal hernia. Surg Endosc. 2013;27:4409–28.
5. Ravi K, Katzka DA. Esophageal impedance monitoring: clinical pearls and pitfalls. Am J Gastroenterol. 2016;111:1245–56.
6. Orlando LA, Orlando RC. Dilated intercellular spaces as a marker of GERD. Curr Gastroenterol Rep. 2009;11:190–4.
7. Dunbar KB, Agoston AT, Odze RD, et al. Association of Acute Gastroesophageal Reflux Disease with Esophageal Histologic Changes. JAMA. 2016;315:2104–12.
8. Muthusamy VR, Lightdale JR, Acosta RD, et al. The role of endoscopy in the management of GERD. Gastrointest Endosc. 2015;81:1305–10.
9. Aziz Q, Fass R, Gyawali CP, et al. Esophageal disorders. Gastroenterology. 2016;150:1368–79.
10. Francis DO, Vaezi MF. Should the reflex be reflux? Throat symptoms and alternative explanations. Clin Gastroenterol Hepatol. 2015;13:1560–6.
11. George N, Abdallah J, Maradey-Romero C, et al. Review article: the current treatment of non-cardiac chest pain. Aliment Pharmacol Ther. 2016;43:213–39.
12. Scarpellini E, Ang D, Pauwels A, et al. Management of refractory typical GERD symptoms. Nat Rev Gastroenterol Hepatol. 2016;13:281–94.
13. Yamasaki T, Fass R. Reflux hypersensitivity: a new functional esophageal disorder. J Neurogastroenterol Motil. 2017;23:495–503.
14. Gyawali CP, Fass R. Management of gastroesophageal reflux disease. Gastroenterology. 2018;154:302–18.

Chapter 12
Functional Esophageal Disorders

Introduction

Patients with functional esophageal disorders present with symptoms suggestive of esophageal disease that are not secondary to GERD, major esophageal motility disorders (achalasia, EGJ outflow obstruction, jackhammer esophagus, distal esophageal spasm, and absent contractility), structural abnormality, or histopathological diagnoses (such as eosinophilic esophagitis). Symptoms must be present for the last 3 months with onset of symptoms at least 6 months prior to diagnosis. Esophageal hypersensitivity, abnormal central processing of peripheral stimuli, autonomic dysregulation, hypervigilance, and psychological comorbidity are some of the proposed mechanisms thought to be important in symptom generation of these patients (see Fig. 12.1) [1]. The current Rome IV classification of functional esophageal disorders includes functional heartburn, reflux hypersensitivity, functional chest pain, functional dysphagia, and globus, each of which will be described in the following sections. The newest iteration of the Rome criteria takes into account esophageal motor disorders, the wide spectrum of symptoms attributable to eosinophilic esophagitis, mechanical obstructions, and the overlap of functional esophageal disorders with GERD.

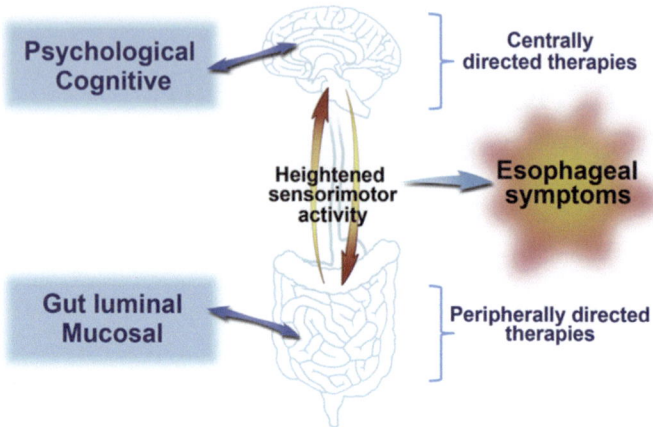

Figure 12.1 The role of the brain-gut axis in mediating esophageal symptoms. Gut luminal and mucosal injury can sensitize visceral afferents causing allodynia or hyperalgesia. Psychological and cognitive factors such as hypervigilance participate in heightened pain perception. Thus, both centrally and peripherally directed treatments can be helpful in management. (With permission from Aziz et al. [1])

Functional Heartburn

Functional heartburn is defined as retrosternal burning pain or discomfort that does not improve with anti-secretory therapy and without evidence of GERD as the underlying cause of symptoms. Prevalence of functional heartburn approximates 50% in PPI non-responders and 25% of non-treated heartburn patients. Proposed mechanisms for heartburn symptom generation include esophageal hypersensitivity (non-painful stimuli are perceived as painful, and painful stimuli are perceived as more painful) due to abnormal peripheral or central processing (anxiety, stress, sleep deprivation, and psychological disorders) of esophageal stimuli. The diagnostic approach in these patients includes an upper endoscopy to evaluate for GERD or other mucosal abnormalities and mucosal biopsies to exclude eosinophilic esophagitis (EoE). If the upper endoscopy is unremarkable, patients with confirmed GERD (positive upper endoscopy or abnormal pH test) will undergo reflux testing, using pH-impedance. In those with no documented history of GERD, the patients should undergo pH testing, preferably by the wireless pH capsule, off treatment. Regardless of the reflux testing, all patients should undergo esophageal manometry to exclude major esophageal motor disorder. Patients with functional heartburn have normal esophageal acid exposure, and no association of symptoms with reflux events (any type). The diagnostic criteria for functional heartburn are the following:

1. Burning retrosternal discomfort or pain.
2. No symptom relief despite optimal anti-secretory therapy.
3. Absence of evidence that gastroesophageal reflux (abnormal acid exposure and symptom reflux association) or eosinophilic esophagitis is the cause of symptoms.
4. Absence of major esophageal motor disorders (achalasia, EGJ outflow obstruction, distal esophageal spasm, jackhammer esophagus and absent peristalsis).

Treatment includes reassurance, neuromodulators, psychological intervention, and alternative/complimentary medicine. Neuromodulators such as tricyclic antidepressants (TCAs) and selective serotine serotonin reuptake inhibitors (SSRIs) are commonly used. Behavioral therapies including cognitive behavioral therapy (CBT), relaxation techniques, mindfulness, and hypnotherapy should be considered as well. Acupuncture may also be helpful as primary or adjunctive therapy.

Reflux Hypersensitivity

Reflux hypersensitivity, formerly termed the hypersensitive esophagus, has been introduced as a new functional esophageal disorder by Rome IV. The diagnostic criteria for reflux hypersensitivity are summarized below:

1. Retrosternal symptoms including heartburn and chest pain.
2. Normal endoscopy and absence of eosinophilic esophagitis as cause of symptoms.
3. Absence of major esophageal motor disorders (achalasia, EGJ outflow obstruction, distal esophageal spasm, jackhammer esophagus, and absent peristalsis).
4. Evidence of triggering of symptoms by reflux events despite normal esophageal acid exposure on pH or pH-impedance monitoring (respond to anti-secretory therapy does not exclude the diagnosis).

In Rome II, reflux hypersensitivity was included in the functional heartburn group. Subsequently, Rome III incorporated these patients into the NERD group. Unlike functional heartburn, there is a higher chance of documenting chronic esophageal histological changes, such as dilated intercellular spaces, papillary elongation, and basal cell elongation, in patients with reflux hypersensitivity. Overlap may exist between reflux hypersensitivity and GERD. Reflux hypersensitivity is estimated to account for 14% of the total patients presenting with heartburn. In a cohort of patients (n = 329) with normal endoscopy who underwent pH-impedance testing, 36% were diagnosed with reflux hypersensitivity, 40% with true NERD, and 24% with functional heartburn. The study also suggested that as compared to a pH test, pH-impedance allows to diagnose more reflux hypersensitivity patients, because it can identify patients who are sensitive to non-acidic reflux.

The diagnostic approach includes an empirical PPI treatment. Reflux hypersensitivity patients may demonstrate complete or partial response to PPI treatment. In patients who present with failure to respond to twice daily PPI, an upper endoscopy is performed to evaluate for mucosal abnormalities. Mucosal biopsies are obtained to exclude eosinophilic esophagitis. If the endoscopy is unremarkable, ambulatory pH testing or wireless pH capsule is performed off PPI therapy to assess for esophageal acid exposure and correlation with reflux events in those with no proven history of

GERD. In patients with documented history of GERD in the past, pH-impedance should be done on PPI treatment. Prior making the diagnosis of reflux hypersensitivity, all patients should undergo high-resolution esophageal manometry to exclude a major esophageal motor disorder.

Failure of PPI treatment in this group of patients usually results in therapy with neuromodulators, because as with other functional esophageal disorders, patients with reflux hypersensitivity demonstrate esophageal hypersensitivity. However, the role of TLESR reducers, endoscopic treatment of GERD, and anti-reflux surgery has yet to be fully elucidated in this patient population.

Functional Chest Pain

Functional chest pain is defined as recurrent, unexplained retrosternal chest pain with negative cardiac workup. The true prevalence of functional chest pain in the general population is not known because population-based surveys assessing noncardiac chest pain did not exclude prior or undiagnosed history of GERD, esophageal motor disorders, or eosinophilic esophagitis. However, the prevalence of functional chest pain appears to be equal between genders, more common in subjects younger than 50 years old and those living in developed countries. All patients presenting with chest pain, even if suspected to be noncardiac, should undergo an evaluation to exclude coronary artery disease by either cardiologist or primary care physician before functional chest pain could be considered. After excluding a cardiac cause, patients should undergo an upper endoscopy to rule out GERD or other mucosal abnormalities and mucosal biopsies to exclude eosinophilic esophagitis. If the test is negative, further workup that includes a pH (off anti-reflux treatment) or pH-impedance test (on anti-reflux treatment) and esophageal manometry should be pursued. Because of the high prevalence of GERD in noncardiac chest pain (NCCP), a high dose of PPI therapy (PPI test) is often initiated to determine whether GERD may be triggering the chest pain symptom. Underlying mechanisms of functional chest pain include abnormal mechano-physical properties of the esophagus (hyperactive and reduced compliance), esophageal hypersensitivity (peripheral and central sensitization), altered autonomic activity, and psychological comorbidity (panic attack, anxiety, and depression).

The Rome IV diagnostic criteria for functional chest pain are the following:

1. Retrosternal chest pain or discomfort (cardiac causes should be ruled out).
2. Absence of associated esophageal symptoms, such as heartburn and dysphagia.
3. Absence of evidence that gastroesophageal reflux or eosinophilic esophagitis is the cause of symptoms.
4. Absence of major esophageal motor disorders (achalasia, EGJ outflow obstruction, distal esophageal spasm, jackhammer esophagus, and absent peristalsis).

Treatment includes neuromodulators such as TCAs, trazodone, SSRIs, serotonin norepinephrine reuptake inhibitors (SNRIs), and others. In addition, psychological interventions such as cognitive behavioral therapy (CBT), hypnosis, and coping skills are becoming more widely accepted as treatment options for functional chest pain.

Functional Dysphagia

Functional dysphagia is defined as the sensation of food sticking, or abnormally passing through the esophagus without objective evidence of esophageal dysmotility, oropharyngeal dysphagia, esophageal mechanical obstruction, or mucosal disease (GERD or eosinophilic esophagitis). Functional dysphagia is estimated to account for 7–8% of the dysphagia patients and represents the least common of all functional esophageal disorders. Diagnostic studies include upper endoscopy with biopsy, pH testing or pH-impedance, esophageal manometry, and barium esophagram with a solid bolus (tablet, cookie, marshmallow) to evaluate for subtle esophageal mucosal abnormalities. Abnormal esophageal sensory perception is considered to be the main underlying mechanism in symptom generation of functional dysphagia patients.

The criteria for functional dysphagia per Rome IV include the following:

1. Sense of solid/liquid foods sticking, lodging, or passing abnormally through the esophagus.
2. Absence of evidence that esophageal mucosal or structural abnormality is the cause of symptoms.
3. Absence of evidence that gastroesophageal reflux or eosinophilic esophagitis is the cause of symptoms.
4. Absence of major esophageal motor disorders (achalasia, EGJ outflow obstruction, distal esophageal spasm, jackhammer esophagus and absent peristalsis).

Often symptoms improve over time and beside reassurance do not require additional therapy. Life style modifications may be sufficient in patients with mild symptoms (small meals, eating in the upright position, lubricating food with dressing, gravy, sauce, or even water and others). Treatment is focused on short trial of PPI therapy to assess whether the dysphagia symptoms may be part of the GERD spectrum. Neuromodulators and empiric esophageal dilation often times with a Maloney dilator (50–54 French dilators) may be considered in more severe cases.

Globus

Globus is defined as a non-painful sensation of fullness or foreign body in the back of the throat, often localized to the sternal notch, that is present without oral intake, and improves with eating and swallowing. Though the actual prevalence of globus is not known, up to 46% of healthy individuals describe events of globus sensation, with peak incidence of symptoms in middle age and without gender predilection. Symptoms continue on for at least 3 years in up to 75% of patients. Underlying pathophysiological mechanisms that may be responsible for symptom generation include esophageal and laryngeal hypersensitivity. Abnormalities in the upper esophageal sphincter complex have not been shown to always correlate with globus symptoms. Diagnostic evaluation of globus includes ruling out structural etiology with a laryngoscopy. If this test is negative, empiric treatment with high-dose PPI for 8 weeks is considered. If the patient responds, globus sensation can be attributed to GERD. If the patient does not respond, an upper endoscopy is required to evaluate for esophageal mucosal abnormalities and specifically for the presence of gastric inlet patch in the proximal esophagus. Patients not responsive to PPI and without other etiologies to explain symptoms are diagnosed with globus. The Rome IV diagnostic criteria are as follow:

1. Persistent or intermittent, non-painful, sensation of a lump or foreign body in the throat with no structural lesion identified on physical examination, laryngoscopy, or endoscopy.

    (a) Occurrence of the sensation between meals.
    (b) Absence of dysphagia or odynophagia.
    (c) Absence of gastric inlet patch in the proximal esophagus.

2. Absence of evidence that gastroesophageal reflux or eosinophilic esophagitis is the cause of symptoms.
3. Absence of major esophageal motor disorders (achalasia, EGJ outflow obstruction, distal esophageal spasm, jackhammer esophagus and absent peristalsis).

The major therapeutic approach to globus remains, reassurance given the benign course of the condition and the high likelihood of having long-term symptoms. Other therapeutic modalities include neuromodulators, psychological intervention, and alternative plus complimentary medicine.

Reference

1. Aziz Q, Fass R, Gyawali CP, et al. Esophageal disorders. Gastroenterology. 2016;150:1368–79.

Chapter 13
Esophageal Injury

Introduction

There are numerous mechanisms that can lead to esophageal mucosal injury where pill-induced injury is likely the most common one. There is a long list of medications that can lead to esophageal mucosa damage. Other esophageal injury disorders include caustic injury, acid- and alkali-induced injury, and radiation esophagitis. AIDS presents an opportunity for various infections to lead to esophageal injury in the context of the immunocompromised patient.

Pill-Induced Injury

Current estimates suggest that more than 70 drugs are capable of causing injury to the esophageal mucosa. Drugs that are commonly associated with pill-induced injury include potassium chloride tablets, tetracycline, doxycycline, quinidine, vitamin C, and alendronate. The injury to the esophageal mucosa may vary from an acute self-limited ulceration to refractory stricture and even death. Mechanisms of pill-induced injury include direct irritant effect of the medication and disruption of the prostaglandin barrier in the stomach and esophagus as noted with NSAIDs and aspirin. The risk of pill-induced injury increases with age. Other factors that increase the risk for pill-induced injury include multiple medications, esophageal structural and motility abnormalities (i.e., left atrial enlargement, recent thoracic surgery), reduced salivary flow, and increased time in the supine position. Females are more likely to have pill-induced injury than males, in a ratio of 2 to 1. Most patients who develop pill-induced injury have no antecedent esophageal injury. The injury to the mucosa is a function of the effects of the drug on the esophagus and the circumstances under which the drug is taken (e.g., while supine and without water).

The common location for pill-induced injury is in the proximal esophagus (at the level of the aortic arch, approximately 23 cm from the incisors). Patients with left atrial enlargement commonly have pill-induced injury at the distal esophagus. Patients typically present with chest pain and odynophagia. Dysphagia, when present, typically reflects inflammatory changes with potential emergence of a stricture. Stricture formation may occur without prior patient complaints. Strictures are more commonly encountered with quinidine, potassium chloride, and alendronate. See Fig. 13.1 for the endoscopic appearance of pill-induced esophageal injury.

Pill-induced injury is often suspected after a careful history. Confirmation of diagnosis can be obtained by endoscopy, which is more sensitive in detecting mucosal changes than radiographic studies. Radiography may be used first if strictures are suspected. Most cases of pill-induced esophagitis will resolve spontaneously within a few weeks. Antacids, H2 blockers, proton pump inhibitors, and sucralfate are commonly used but are of unproven benefit. Management of pill-induced strictures may be difficult, requiring repeated esophageal dilations.

Prevention is best obtained by educating both health-care professionals and patients that medications should be taken with at least 150 mL of water (250 mL if using alendronate) prior to and during pill consumption. In addition, prescribing the medication in liquid form can be helpful. The patient should be instructed to take all pills while upright and to

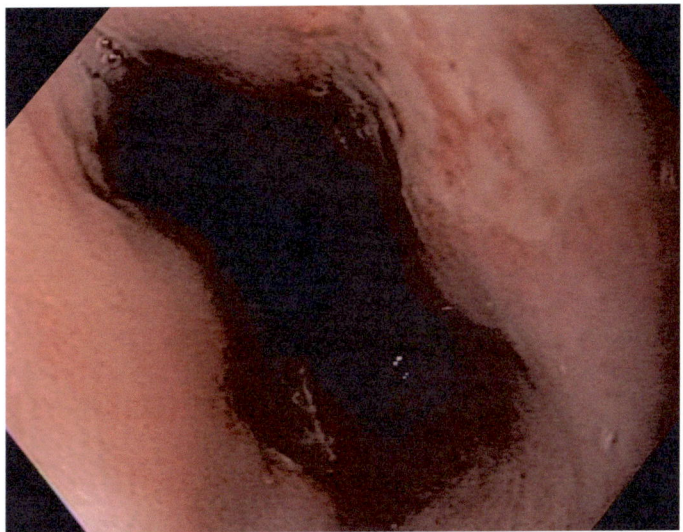

FIGURE 13.1 Pill-induced esophagitis. Patient presented to upper endoscopy with symptoms of dysphagia after taking several doses of NSAIDs without fluid

remain in this position for at least 15 min (30 min if using alendronate).

Caustic Injury

Caustic injury is most commonly encountered in the pediatric population, with over half of cases occurring in children <5 years old. These cases are nearly always due to accidental ingestion. In adolescents and adults, caustic ingestion occurs under the influence of drugs, in patients with mental illness, or in those who attempt to commit suicide. Severity and extent of caustic injury to the esophagus are dependent on the following characteristics: alkaline vs acidic properties of the ingested substance; the quantity, concentration, and composition of the substance (liquid vs solid); and length of time of substance contact with esophageal mucosa. Of all chemicals that can be ingested, strong alkali and acids are most likely to result in injury, with alkaline materials more likely to affect the esophageal mucosa.

Acid-Induced Injury

Acids produce coagulative necrosis in the esophagus. They pass rapidly through the esophagus, and the superficial necrosis produced is thought to be protective to the esophageal mucosa. Strong acids are more likely to produce injury to the stomach, although clinically significant esophageal burns may occur in less than half the patients.

Alkali-Induced Injury

Alkaline materials include sodium or potassium hydroxide chemicals, detergents, and button batteries. They produce liquefaction necrosis and result in rapid and deep esophageal and gastric injury and usually lasts for 3–4 days with the development of focal to extensive sloughing and ulceration of the mucosa and later development of granulation tissue and fibrosis over weeks. Full thickness burns are not uncommon. The degree of signs and symptoms does not accurately predict the level of injury. In adults, especially when suicide is the underlying motive, multiple agents should be suspected. Consequently, the clinical presentation may be quite variable, ranging from no symptoms to evidence of mediastinitis, cardiovascular collapse, and death.

Initial management includes assessment of airway patency and breathing. Since the respiratory tract may be involved. Patients should be assessed for hemodynamic instability, and, if present, fluids and blood products should be considered. Unstable patients should be managed in the intensive care unit. There is no role for removing the caustic agent by lavage via nasogastric tubes, inducing vomiting or neutralizing the substance. All these attempts may cause further injury. Thereafter, upper endoscopy should be performed within 12–24 h. The absence of any signs or symptoms does not exclude severe foregut injury. Endoscopy should be avoided in patients suspected of esophageal perforation.

The subsequent proposed grading system with associated management is a reflection of the degree of esophageal injury and predicted clinical outcomes.

Grade 0: Normal.
Grade I: Mucosal edema, hyperemia.
Grade II: Ulcers; superficial ulcers, exudates, bleeding (IIA), deep focal ulcers (IIB).
Grade III: Necrosis; focal (IIIA), extensive (IIIB).

Grades I and IIA patients have excellent prognosis with little risk of subsequent stricture formation. Patients with greater than Grade IIB injury have more than 70% likelihood of stricture formation, with some patients requiring surgical intervention. The use of corticosteroids aiming to reduce stricture formation is controversial and is currently not recommended in the setting of advanced grade injury. Broad spectrum antibiotics have been considered a standard of care in patient with Grade III injury and suspicion for esophageal perforation. Proton pump inhibitors may be useful in preventing superimposed GERD, and this may be required for several months until healing has occurred. The timing of esophageal dilation for ingestion-associated strictures also remains the subject of disagreement. Some authors recommend initiating dilation with small dilators once the patient is stabilized, hoping to keep the lumen open. Early dilation is generally not recommended due to increased risk of perforation. Most practitioners will wait 3–6 days post ingestion for dilation consideration. Repeated dilation of resistant stricture is a long-term consequence of caustic injury.

Radiation Esophagitis

Radiation esophagitis occurs in 50% of patients receiving radiotherapy to the thorax or head and neck region. Radiation suppresses cell proliferation at the basal layer of the epithelium. These cells usually recover in a few days, but repeated radiation will lead to permanent cell damage. Furthermore, radiation can cause thrombosis of blood vessels, leading to ischemia, tissue necrosis, and ulcer formation. Symptoms of acute radiation-induced injury include chest pain, dysphagia, and odynophagia, which begin to manifest during the second week of radiation exposure. These symptoms can be confused with candida esophagitis, which also commonly occurs as a result of radiation treatment. Chronic radiation-induced esophageal injury is associated with inflammation and fibrosis formation within the esophageal musculature and is seen 3–6 months after radiation therapy completion. Symptoms and findings of chronic radiation injury include dysphagia-related esophageal stricture, esophageal dysmotility, ulceration, tracheoesophageal fistula, and esophageal perforation.

Treatment for acute radiation esophagitis includes supportive measures such as dietary modifications, viscous lidocaine, treatment of concomitant candida esophagitis, and nutritional support. The radiation dose should be decreased by 10%, or the radiotherapy should be interrupted temporarily. The formation of stricture requires endoscopic dilation or gastrostomy feeding.

Esophageal Injury in the Immunocompromised Patient

AIDS

In the past, esophageal involvement was commonly encountered in AIDS patients. In the early days of the disease, many patients presented with Candida esophagitis. The use of highly active antiretroviral treatment (HAART) has resulted in a reduction in the frequency of opportunistic infections in AIDS patients. These infections typically occur when the CD4 count is <200 per mm^3. However, in the era of HAART, it is now more common for AIDS patients to complain of esophageal symptoms not specific to AIDS.

Candida still remains the most common cause of esophageal infection in patients with AIDS and those with primary HIV infection, the latter of which is related to the transient immunosuppression occurring with initial infection (Fig. 13.2). Patients complain of symptoms of substernal chest pain with dysphagia. The presence of oral thrush predicts concomitant esophageal candidiasis; however, the absence of thrush does not rule out the presence of esophageal candidiasis. Cytomegalovirus has also been associated with esophageal ulcerations with characteristic symptoms of odynophagia and severe substernal chest pain with findings of large deep ulcerations in the esophagus. Herpes simplex-associated esophageal ulcerations are associated with diffuse shallow ulcerations in the esophagus. In patients with advanced AIDS with CD4 count <50 mm^3, idiopathic aphthous ulcerations can be encountered in the esophagus with very similar endoscopic findings related to CMV. Esophageal ulcerations that are observed on endoscopy require exclusion of Kaposi's sarcoma, lymphoma, squamous cell carcinoma, adenocarcinoma, and pill-induced injury (e.g., zidovudine and zalcitabine).

Endoscopy is key to evaluate symptomatic patients with AIDS and is indicated for those patients who fail to improve with empiric antifungal therapy for esophageal candidiasis. Those suspected of having *Candida* infection should be treated empirically with fluconazole 100 mg once daily for 2 weeks after a loading dose of 200 mg. CMV and HSV esophageal ulcers should be treated with antibiotics; CMV, ganciclovir 5 mg/kg dose every 12 h until oral therapy is tolerated for 3–6 weeks, and HSV, acyclovir 400 mg, five times daily for 14–21 days. Idiopathic aphthous ulcer-

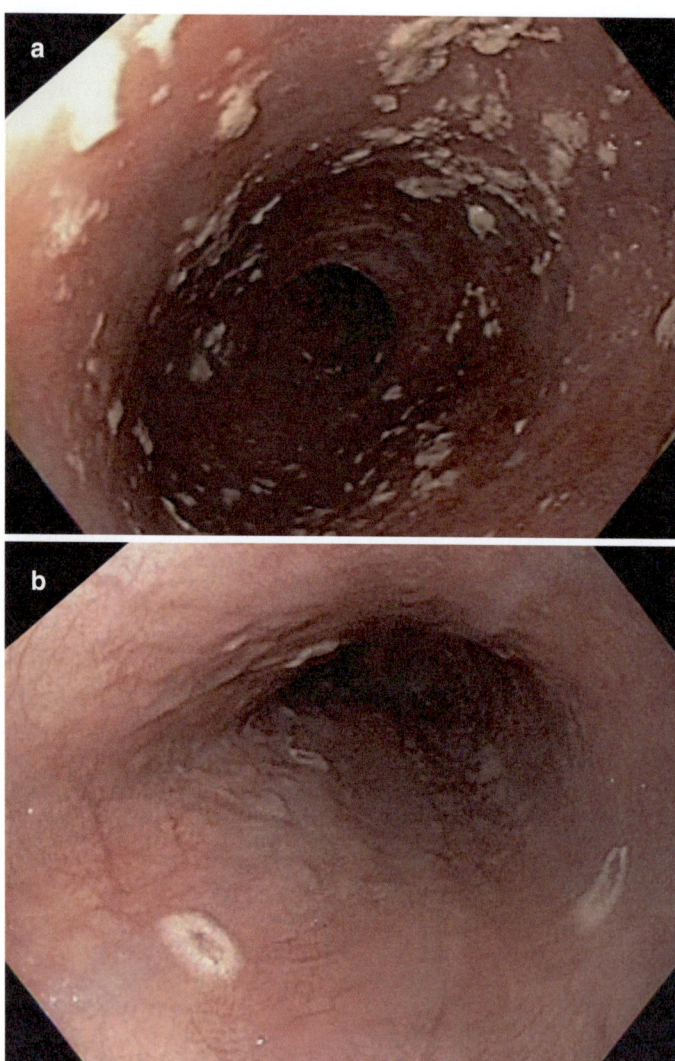

FIGURE 13.2 Endoscopic appearance of candida esophagitis. Both AIDS patients reported symptoms of dysphagia and odynophagia over the last few weeks. (**a**) Cheesy white exudates of *Candida albicans* typical of candida esophagitis. (**b**) Small discrete white appearing ulcers noted throughout the esophagus with biopsies consistent with *Candida albicans*

ations respond well to oral steroids with tapering over a period of 4 weeks. Patients who are not responsive to steroids can be treated with thalidomide as a second-line agent.

Suggested Reading

1. Fass R. Pill esophagitis. Curr Treat Opt Gastroenterol. 2000;3:89–93.

Chapter 14
Graft Versus Host Disease

The esophagus may be affected during the course of bone marrow transplantation. Both chemotherapy and radiotherapy may cause injury to the esophageal mucosa. Additionally, patients are immunocompromised and thus are more susceptible to various infections. Finally, graft-versus-host disease (GVHD) may develop. Both acute and chronic forms may occur. In the acute form, all portions of the gastrointestinal tract may be injured, leading to more general gastrointestinal symptoms. Diarrhea is the most common symptom, followed by anorexia, dyspepsia, food intolerance, nausea, and vomiting. Acute esophageal GVHD may present as vesiculobullous, ulcerative, or desquamative lesions. Chronic GVHD may also occur, and if present in the esophagus, it may result in proximal esophageal strictures or webs. Patient may complain of dysphagia, and esophageal dilation may be required.

Suggested Reading

1. McDonald GB, Sullivan KM, Schuffler MD, et al. Esophageal abnormalities in chronic graft-versus-host disease in humans. Gastroenterology. 1981;80(5 pt 1):914–21.

Chapter 15
Eosinophilic Esophagitis (EoE)

Introduction

Eosinophilic esophagitis (EoE) was originally described in the pediatric population but in the last two decades has been increasingly recognized in adults. It is a chronic inflammatory process defined by esophageal symptoms, a dense eosinophilic epithelial infiltration (>15 eosinophils/HPF), and the absence of other etiologies causing esophageal eosinophilia. The prevalence of EoE in the United States is estimated to be approximately 57 per 100,000 persons. EoE is an immune-mediated disease by which environmental and food antigens stimulate the Th2 inflammatory cascade.

Clinical Presentation

Children present with symptoms of abdominal pain, vomiting, heartburn, and chest pain with associated food impaction that may be related to underlying esophageal stricture or narrowing. Adults, on the other hand, more frequently (30–80%) present with food impaction but most commonly present with dysphagia as well as heartburn, chest pain, nausea, and other symptoms. Interestingly the degree of mucosal eosinophilia does not correlate with dysphagia severity or symptom improvement with treatment. The degree of dysphagia is more likely related to other factors such as concomitant esophageal dysmotility, degree of mucosal inflammation, and fibrostenosis.

Diagnosis

The two phenotypes of EoE are defined as the inflammatory and fibrostenotic type (see Table 15.1 for comparison of features) [1]. Additional histological features used to support the diagnosis of EoE include eosinophilic degranulation, eosinophilic microabscesses, extension of epithelium into mucosal layers (rete peg elongation), basal zone hyperplasia, spongiosis (intercellular dilation), and fibrosis of the lamina propria. Endoscopic findings may include uniform small-caliber esophagus, single or multiple corrugations, esophageal furrows, mucosal abscesses, and a stricture. See Fig. 15.1 for a typical endoscopic appearance of eosinophilic esophagitis.

Diagnosis is established after biopsies demonstrate dense eosinophilic infiltrate (>15 eosinophils per high-power field). Due to the patchy nature of the eosinophilic infiltrate, two to

TABLE 15.1 Phenotypes of eosinophilic esophagitis (EoE). The two major phenotypes of EoE with description of endoscopic appearance and recommended treatments for symptoms

	Endoscopic appearance	**Treatments with good outcomes**
Inflammatory phenotype	Pale mucosa, decreased vascularity, white exudate, longitudinal furrows	Oral steroids or elimination diet
Fibrostenotic phenotype	Transient (feline) and fixed rings, narrow caliber esophagus, fragile esophageal mucosal appearance ("crepe-paper mucosa")	Esophageal dilation

With permission from Richter et al. [1]

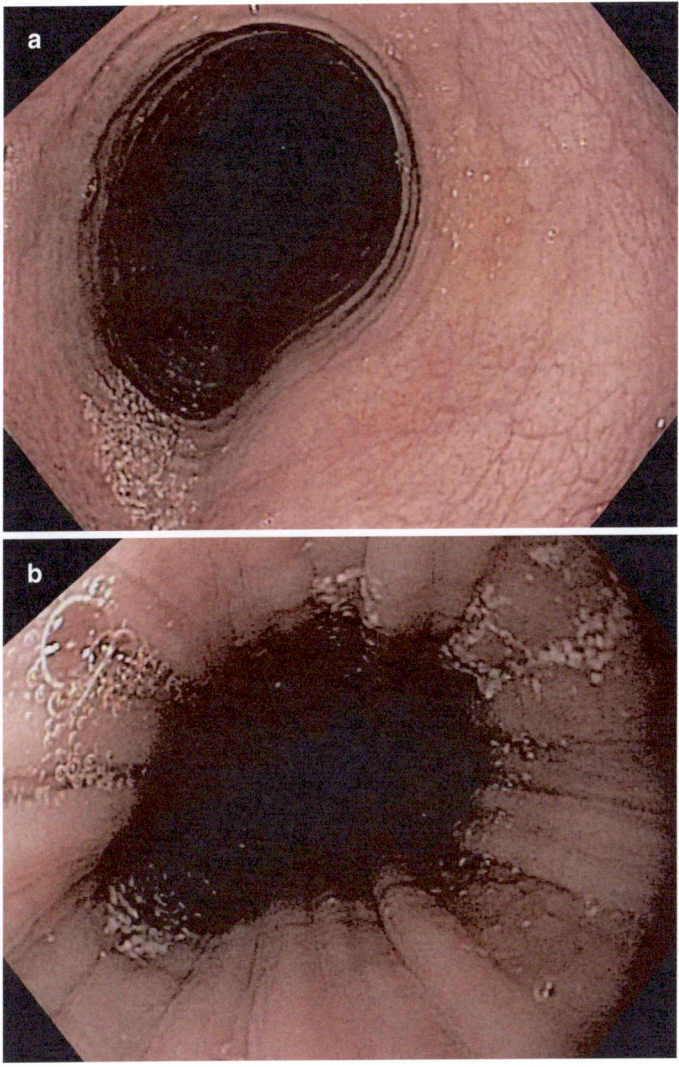

FIGURE 15.1 Endoscopic appearances of eosinophilic esophagitis. (a) Felinization and furrowing of the esophagus in eosinophilic esophagitis. (b) Microabscesses of eosinophilic esophagitis

four biopsies are taken from the distal and proximal esophagus during endoscopy to confirm the diagnosis. Esophageal tear may occur after simple passage of the endoscope, during biopsy, or after dilation. Esophageal manometry findings in EoE include panpressurization, which is also seen in achalasia, and increased intrabolus pressure. The role of GERD in EoE remains controversial, and pH testing is not routinely done in these patients, as pH profiles do not predict PPI response. Overall, 50–80% of children, and to a lesser extent in adults, have concomitant allergic disease such as allergic rhinitis, asthma, and food allergy. A referral to an allergist may be prudent in these patients to test for associated allergic conditions given the complex interplay of these conditions. A positive allergy test for a particular food may identify food as an underlying cause for EoE.

Management

The management goals for EoE include improvement of symptoms, especially dysphagia and fear of food impactions, histological remission of esophageal eosinophilia, endoscopic treatment for eosinophilic inflammation or strictures, and prevention of long-term complications such as strictures, diffuse esophageal narrowing, and food impactions. The first step in the treatment of EoE includes high-dose PPI trial followed by endoscopic assessment of response to therapy including repeat biopsies to assess the eosinophilic infiltrate of the mucosa. This helps to differentiate patients who have GERD-related eosinophilia, PPI-responsive esophageal eosinophilia (PPI-REE), and EoE. Patients who have significant drop in eosinophilic infiltrate on PPI therapy, decreased inflammation and symptoms in the absence of objective evidence of GERD, are re-categorized as PPI-REE. In those with EoE, treatments include topical steroids such as aerosolized fluticasone as well as budesonide respules or slurry, twice daily.

Complications of treatment include oral candidiasis, which occurs in approximately 1% of patients. Both treatments have been shown to decrease eosinophilic infiltrates, but with less impressive symptom response. If topical steroids are stopped after initial treatment, most patients will relapse. Thus, maintenance therapy is often required for most patients. Other therapies that have been evaluated in EoE in a few studies include montelukast, a leukotriene inhibitor, azathioprine, IL-5 inhibitors, (mepolizumab and reslizumab), and anti-IgE antibody (omalizumab). In addition, dietary restrictions have been used in EoE as a long-term treatment modality for patients who can sustain such regimens as elemental diet, six food elimination diet (SFED), and targeted elimination diet. These diets demonstrated varying degrees of successes (40–90% with the highest being in patients taking elemental diets). Lastly, in some patients with a clear fibrostenotic disease, esophageal dilation with either a Savary or Maloney esophageal dilator for symptomatic relief has been recommended.

Reference

1. Richter JE. Current Management of Eosinophilic Esophagitis 2015. J Clin Gastroenterol. 2016;50:99–110.

Chapter 16
Other Esophageal Disorders

Other disorders in which the esophagus may be involved include Behcet's syndrome, in which erosions or ulcerations may be present. Typically, the ileum and colon are involved in these patients. Gastrointestinal involvement is a minor criterion for the diagnosis of Behcet's syndrome. Patients with amyloidosis may have esophageal involvement. Radiographic and manometric involvement can be much more frequent than symptoms referable to amyloid deposition.

Cowden's syndrome is an autosomal dominant disease associated with breast and thyroid cancer with notable mucocutaneous ulcerations. Benign polyps, hamartomas, are found throughout the gastrointestinal tract in 70–85% of patients. These hamartomas may be seen in the esophagus but are more commonly found in the colon. Glycogenic acanthosis also has been described in the esophagus of these patients.

Suggested Reading

1. Ideguchi H, Suda A, Takeno M, et al. Gastrointestinal Manifestations of Bechet's disease in Japan: a study of 43 patients. Rheumatol Int. 2014;34:851–6.

Index

A
Acanthosis nigricans (AN), 44
Achalasia
  Chagas disease, 22
  description, 21
  endoscopic appearance, 23
  esophageal manometry, 24
  esophagectomy, 29
  Heller myotomy, 79
  neuronal denervation, 22
  peroral endoscopic myotomy, 29
  pneumatic dilation, 28
  radiographs, 24
  secondary, 29–30
  symptom, 22
  treatment, 25
Acid-induced injury, 136
Acute radiation-induced injury, 138
Adenocarcinoma
  Barrett's esophagus, 53
  diagnosis, 53
  endoscopic appearance, 53
  hoarseness, 52
  incidence, 52
Alkali-induced injury, 136
Ambulatory 24-h esophageal pH monitoring, GERD, 102
Amyloidosis, 151
Anti-reflux surgery, 116
Aortic arch, 75

B
Barium esophagram, 63
Barrett's esophagus, 52–58
Bazex syndrome, 44
Behcet's syndrome, 151
Benign epithelial tumors, 59
Benign polyps, 151
Bravo test, 103
Bullous skin disease, esophageal involvement, 41

C
Candida albicans, 140
Candida infection in AIDS patients, 139
Carcinosarcoma, 58
Caustic ingestion, 135
Cervical web, 65
Chagas disease, 22
Chemotherapy, 143
Chronic cough, PPI therapy, 106
Chronic PPI treatment, adverse effects of, 115
Chronic radiation-induced esophageal injury, 138

Cicatricial pemphigoid (CP), 42
Collagen vascular disease, 45–46
Cowden's syndrome, 151
Cricopharyngeus muscle, 4

D
Dermatomyositis, 45
Dilated intercellular spaces (DIS), 95–97
Distal contractile integral (DCI) measures, 20
Distal esophageal spasm (DES), 34–35
Diverticulum
  epiphrenic, 71
  mid-esophageal
    diverticula, 68
    traction, 70
  Zenker's, 67
Duodenogastroesophageal reflux, 93–94
Dysphagia, 59, 67
  description, 11
  diverticulum (*see* Diverticulum)
  eosinophilic esophagitis, 146
  esophageal, 14, 15
  graft-versus-host disease, 143
  lower esophageal ring, 63
  lusoria, 75
  oropharyngeal, 11, 13
Dysplasia, 56–57

E
Endoscopic mucosal resection (EMR) technique, 51
Endoscopy, dysphagia, 49
Enteric nervous system, 5
Eosinophilic esophagitis (EoE)
  clinical presentation, 145
  description, 145
  diagnosis, 146–148
  dietary restrictions, 149
  elemental diet, 149
  management goals, 148
  phenotypes, 146
  prevalence, 145
  six food elimination diet, 149
  targeted elimination diet, 149
  topical steroids treatment, 148
Epidermolysis bullosa (EB), 41–43
Epidermolysis bullosa acquisita (EBA), 42
Epiphrenic diverticula, 71
Erosive esophagitis (EE), 86
  classification systems for, 101
  upper endoscopy, 100
Esophageal dysmotility, 90
Esophageal dysphagia, 14–15
Esophageal intramural pseudodiverticulosis, 72, 73
Esophageal manometry, 17
Esophageal motility disorders, 70
  absent contractility, 30–34
  achalasia, 21–29
  Chicago Classification, v3.0, 17–20
  distal esophageal spasm, 34
  EGJ outflow obstruction, 35, 36
  high-resolution esophageal manometry, 17, 26, 38
  ineffective esophageal motility, 36
  Jackhammer esophagus, 34
  mixed connective tissue, 39
  polymyositis, 39
  progressive systemic sclerosis, 37–39
Esophageal mucosal injury, 133
  acid-induced injury, 136
  in AIDS patients, 138, 141
  alkali-induced injury, 136–137
  caustic injury, 135
  pill-induced injury, 133–135
Esophageal syndromes, 85
Esophageal webs, 63, 65, 66
Esophagectomy, 29, 44

Esophagogastric junction (EGJ) outflow obstruction, 35, 36
Esophagus, 1
  anatomy, 3–6
  fishbone, 80, 81
  physiology of swallowing, 6–7
Extra-esophageal syndromes, 85, 106–110

F
Foreign bodies
  body packing, 82, 83
  description, 77
  food impaction, 78–80
  management, 78
  pediatric population, 77
  round foreign bodies, in children, 80
  sharp foreign bodies, 80
  special circumstances, 78
  unique foreign bodies, 80
Functional chest pain, 127–128
Functional dysphagia, 128–129
Functional heartburn, 124–125

G
Gastric dysmotility, 98
Gastroesophageal reflux disease (GERD)
  adverse effects of chronic PPI treatment, 115
  ambulatory 24-h esophageal pH monitoring, 101–103
  anti-reflux barrier, dysfunction of, 89
  anti-reflux surgery, 116
  anti-reflux treatment, 100
  Barrett's esophagus, 53, 54
  defined, 88
  diagnostic evaluation, 100
  dilated intercellular spaces, 95, 96
  double-dose PPI, 94
  duodenogastroesophageal reflux, 93
  endoscopic therapy, 116
  esophageal dysmotility, 90–93
  esophageal hypersensitivity, 98
  extra-esophageal syndromes, 106
  gastric acid secretion, 93
  gastric dysmotility, 98
  genetic factors, 99
  H. pylori infection, 99
  heartburns, 100
  hiatal hernia, 90, 91
  LINX procedure, 116
  management, 113–115
  manifestations and complications, 87
  Montreal classification, 85, 86
  mucosal impedance, 105
  multichannel intraluminal pH impedance, 104
  non-acidic reflux, 94
  noncardiac chest pain, 111–113
  pathophysiological mechanisms, 88, 89
  phenotypes, 85–88
  reflux hypersensitivity in refractory heartburn patients, 118
  refractory heartburn patients, 117–121
  Stretta procedure, 117
  symptoms, 100
  transoral incisionless fundoplication, 117
  upper endoscopy, 100
Gastrointestinal stromal tumors, 60
Gastrointestinal tract, esophageal neoplasia, 47
Gene mapping studies, in GERD patients, 99
Globus, 129–131

Glycogenic acanthosis, 151
Graft-versus-host disease (GVHD), 143
Granular cell tumors, 60

H
Hailey-Hailey disease, 43
Hamartomas, 151
Helicobacter pylori
   eradication, 93
   infection, 99
Heller myotomy, 29, 79
Herpes simplex-associated esophageal ulcerations, 139
Herpes simplex virus (HSV), 43
Hiatal hernia, 90, 91
Highly active antiretroviral treatment (HAART), 139
High-resolution esophageal manometry (HRM), 17–21, 26, 38
Hyperkeratosis plantaris et palmaris, 44
Hyperkeratosis, skin disease, 43–45

I
Ineffective esophageal motility (IEM), 36–37
Iron deficiency anemia, 65

J
Jackhammer esophagus, 34

L
Laryngeal pathologies, 106
Laryngopharyngeal pathologies, 107–109
Leiomyoma, 60

Lower esophageal ring, 63
Lower esophageal sphincter, 5, 7
Lymphoma, 60

M
Malignant melanoma, 58
Mid-esophageal diverticula, 68–71
Mixed connective tissue (MCT) disease, 39
Mucosal impedance (MI), 105
Multichannel intraluminal pH impedance, 103–105
Muscular ring, 63

N
Noncardiac chest pain (NCCP), 111, 113
Nonerosive reflux disease (NERD), 86
   PPI therapy, 114
Nutcracker esophagus, 34

O
Oropharyngeal dysphagia, 11–14

P
Paterson-Kelly syndrome, 65
Pemphigus vulgaris (PV), 42
Peristalsis, 6, 36–37
Peroral endoscopic myotomy (POEM), 111
   achalasia, 29
pH-impedance testing, 105
Pill-induced injury, 133, 135
Plummer-Vinson syndrome, 65
Polymyositis, esophageal motility disorders, 39
PPI therapy, 110
   GERD-related NCCP, 111

PPI-responsive esophageal
eosinophilia
(PPI-REE), 148
Progressive systemic sclerosis
(PSS), 37

R
Rabeprazole, 112
Radiation esophagitis, 138
Radiotherapy, 143
Reflux hypersensitivity, 125–127
Rome IV classification, of
functional esophageal
disorders, 123
functional chest pain, 127
functional dysphagia, 128
functional heartburn, 124
globus, 129
reflux hypersensitivity, 125

S
Schatzki's ring, 63, 64
Scleroderma, 37, 45
Sertraline, 112
Six food elimination diet
(SFED), 149
Small-cell carcinoma, 58
Spinal afferents, 8
Squamous cell carcinoma
(SCC), 44
clinical practice, 48
diagnosis, 49
endoscopic appearance, 49, 50
incidence, 48
treatment, 50
Squamous papilloma, 59, 60
Stevens-Johnson syndrome, 43

Stretta procedure, 117
Subclavian artery, 75
Swallowing
dysphagia, 11
esophagus, 6
Symptom association probability
(SAP) scores, 103
Symptom index (SI), 103

T
Targeted elimination diet, 149
Traction diverticula, 70
Transient lower esophageal
sphincter relaxation
(TLESR), 7, 88, 90
Transoral incisionless
fundoplication
(TIF), 117
Trypanosoma cruzi, 22

U
Ulcerations
in Behcet's syndrome, 151
mucocutaneous, 151
Upper endoscopy, 100
Upper esophageal sphincter, 3, 6

V
Vagal afferents, 8
Venlafaxine, 112
Verrucous carcinoma, 58

Z
Zenker's diverticulum, 67–69

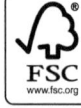

MIX
Papier aus verantwortungsvollen Quellen
Paper from responsible sources
FSC® C105338

If you have any concerns about our products,
you can contact us on
ProductSafety@springernature.com

In case Publisher is established outside the EU,
the EU authorized representative is:
**Springer Nature Customer Service Center GmbH
Europaplatz 3, 69115 Heidelberg, Germany**

Printed by Libri Plureos GmbH
in Hamburg, Germany